Expectations of Recovery
ICU Anecdotes

Gnan Thakore, MD

Publisher:
Pulmonary & Critical Care Consultant Inc.
1520 S. Main #2
Dayton, Ohio 45409
www.pulcare.com

Supported by educational organization:
Heart Health Now
3484 Rockview Rd.
Springfield, Ohio 45504
www.healthnowbooks.com

ISBN: 0999113208
ISBN 13: 9780999113202
Library of Congress Control Number: 2017946112
Pulmonary & Critical Care Consultants Inc
Dayton, Ohio

Gnan Thakore, MD
Associate Clinical Professor of Medicine
Boonshoft School of Medicine
Wright State University
Dayton, Ohio

Director
Medical Intensive Care Unit
Miami Valley Hospital
Dayton, Ohio

Staff Physician
LifeCare Hospitals
Long Term Acute Care Hospital
Dayton, Ohio

2017

Dedicated to my parents,
Narendra Thakore and Jyotsna Thakore

Medical Information Disclaimer

1. Credit
1.1 This document was created using a template from SEQ Legal (http://www.seqlegal.com).
2. No advice
2.1 Our book contains general medical information.
2.2 The medical information is not advice and should not be treated as such.
3. No warranties
3.1 The medical information in this book is provided without any representations or warranties, express or implied.
3.2 Without limiting the scope of Section 3.1, we do not warrant or represent that the medical information in this book
    a) is complete or accurate, as this information is intended only to provide background for the story or
    b) helps with decisions regarding aggressive care in your particular case.

4.   Medical assistance

4.1 You must not rely on the information in this book as an alternative to medical advice from your doctor or other professional health care provider.

4.2 If you have any specific questions about any medical matter, you should consult your doctor or other professional health care provider.

4.3 If you think you may be suffering from any medical condition, you should seek immediate medical attention.

4.4 You should never delay seeking medical advice, disregard medical advice, or discontinue medical treatment because of information in this book.

5.   Limits upon exclusions of liability

5.1 Nothing in this disclaimer will limit any liabilities in any way that is not permitted under applicable law.

Contents

Table of Figures

Acknowledgments

I am very grateful to my wife, Falguni Thakore, a methodical physical therapist, for all her support. She removes all hurdles in my life. I appreciate my sister, Dr. Jigna Thakore, my perpetual cheerleader and a well-loved gastroenterologist. I thank Deborah Hurst and Pamela Lamb, palliative care nurses extraordinaire, for looking over the material and making helpful suggestions. I recognize Dr. Thomas Donnelly, a passionate critical care physician, for making crucial recommendations. Dr. Michael Craig, the founder of our group, and Dr. Vipul Patel, my colleague, read the work and provided encouragement. Anna Schneider provided a family's perspective. Patricia edited and organized the book. Finally, I am grateful to Dr. Glen Solomon, our department chair, for reviewing the book and providing a foreword.

Foreword

Even after forty years in medicine, I find the ICU a wondrous and frightening place. The patients are incredibly sick people, with a bewildering array of physical dysfunctions, metabolic abnormalities, and cognitive impairments. The physicians, nurses, therapists, and care team offer therapies once only dreamt about in science fiction. But despite the technical wonders of intensive care unit care, recovery from major trauma or severe illness is not guaranteed. Furthermore, recovery from an acute event does not guarantee return to presickness level of function, improvement in any underlying condition, or return to good health.

While invasive monitoring and high-tech therapies often constitute the image of the modern ICU, it is the human interaction that defines the ICU experience. Questions to be answered include the following: Who should get intensive care? What is the likelihood of recovery? What care does the patient want? What care does the family want for the patient? When should care be stopped? What constitutes a "good" death?

Dr. Gnan Thakore is an experienced critical care physician, associate clinical professor of medicine, and director of the Medical Intensive Care Unit at Miami Valley Hospital. He brings his years of experience together in a series of case vignettes that provides the reader with insight into the management of critically ill patients. He emphasizes the interpersonal interactions that determine the critical decision-making process. This is not a book about the technical wizardry of modern medicine. It is a primer on how families and patients can make the right medical choices for themselves.

If there is one take-home message from this book, it is that families and friends must have discussions about topics on end-of-life care, quality of life, and personal wishes and desires. These discussions cannot wait until people are elderly, sick, or injured; they should occur when people are of sound mind and mental capacity. This book teaches us that each of us has the power to determine the type of medical care that we want to receive, if only we share our wishes with our loved ones and physicians. It is still the personal contact and the physician-patient interaction that define the "care" in intensive care.

I urge you to read this book and then prepare a living will and appoint a health care power of attorney. Sit down with your spouse, children, family, and friends and tell them your wishes should you become critically ill or injured. Do it today.

Glen D. Solomon, M.D.
Chair, Department of Internal Medicine
Boonshoft School of Medicine, Wright State University

Introduction

We are generally in control of our health care. We decide when we go to the dentist or the doctor, take medications of our own free will, and consent to a surgery. We are in control—until we are unable to make such decisions for ourselves, as in an emergency. An intensive care unit is a place where we go when we are critically ill and where complex decisions need to be made on our behalf, and yet we are often unable to communicate our wishes for care. At this stage, we must leave the decision making to our caregivers and kin.

An important consideration at such times is that our loved ones may not think as we do or know our wishes. Family members may be very emotional and unable to think the problem through. They will try their best to make proper choices in an emergency, but they can only make decisions that are consistent with our wishes if we have discussed our preferences with them.

Occasionally, the choice for aggressive care is a matter of hope, while at other times it is honoring loved one's wishes. Often the decision maker misinterprets patient wishes.

Everyone has a different attitude towards end-of-life care. Most people don't want to be in a vegetative state for any length of time. In America, more people want to be at home when they die, yet a majority die in hospitals; a significant number of these hospitalized patients die in intensive care units.

I would like to share some down-to-earth stories in this book with the hope that they will help people become realistic consumers of intensive care unit care. The aim of the book is straightforward: to provide a brief overview of common illnesses and to discuss how these illnesses impact patients' long-term survival. This book also explains how health care providers interpret patient desires during critical illness. The book will shed light on the intensive care unit experience and what issues *influence* next-of-kin decisions. It will answer questions regarding right use of aggressive care and why it is wise to let your family know your wishes.

A majority of patients in the intensive care unit get better and transfer out; however, many have chronic diseases that bring them back to the hospital. Patients come to a hospital with the expectation of getting better. Modern medicine has set high expectations for recovery from illness. *Balancing high expectations with reality, we consider two groups of patients that don't do well in an ICU: those struck by sudden overwhelming illnesses and those with incurable life-limiting illnesses.* To illustrate these groups, stories are divided among four sections.

Section-one poses some difficult questions as it summarizes the issues explored in this book. Section-three deals with the terminal condition. These two sections constitute the core of our complex topic. The other two sections complete the goals of the book. Section-two discusses common catastrophic illnesses which may either improve or progress to a terminal condition. We focus on brain injuries because patients frequently lose decision-making ability, and at the same time the complexity of recovery evokes many questions and concerns for the family. Section-four illustrates common chronic illnesses/organ failure scenarios that can linger, or advance to a terminal condition. None of the stories fall neatly into one section. Sections are just created to focus on an idea. I encourage you to carefully review the mechanism of illness, prognostication of recovery, as well as human interactions in each of these stories to understand the utility of aggressive care.

All of the anecdotes in this book are true stories, but the names and, occasionally, genders of patients and family members have been changed. Each patient is unique, and these are but a few representative stories out of thousands. The stories have been selected based on the unique issues they raise for discussion, and some stories end with an explanation. I share the story of my father, Naru, in chapter 4.

Statistics change over time, and therefore are not a major focus of this book. The picture of intensive care unit decision-making, however, should remain accurate for the foreseeable future.

Gnan Thakore, MD

Section 1

WHAT IS AGGRESSIVE CARE?

One

Declaration of living will

Since our stories are about complex cases where death is a possibility, we should start by taking a look at the so-called advance directive documents. An advance health care directive is a document drawn up to provide instructions for future care. The most common ones are the living will and the health care power of attorney (or durable power of attorney for health care).

Here are some excerpts from a living will declaration similar to those found in the states of Illinois and Ohio:

I, (full name), being of sound mind, of my free will declare that my moment of death shall not be artificially postponed.

There are two important aspects of a living will, which are as follows:

1. There must be an affirmation that one is in control of his or her mind. A proper living will requires that one can think clearly. It can't be created when decision-making capacity is impaired.
2. There must be a declaration of the finality of the moment of death. The end of life should not be prolonged and postponed by artificial technology:

Do not extend my life if:
I am judged to have an incurable and irreversible injury, disease, or illness resulting in a terminal condition.

Here, the attending physician has determined that death is imminent except for death-delaying procedures. At this stage:

all interventions that would only prolong the dying process should be withheld or withdrawn, and I should be permitted to die naturally. At that stage, only administer medication or perform any medical procedure deemed necessary by my attending physician to provide me with comfort care.

Some states specifically mention "coma state" separately:

If my attending physician and a specialist determine that I am in a permanent coma, then do not administer any life-sustaining treatments. If life-sustaining treatments are underway, that is, if I am already on life support or other aggressive support when the above determination is made, then discontinue all such support.

A "do not resuscitate" (DNR) order should be placed on the chart. DNR orders tell hospital personnel not to perform cardiopulmonary resuscitation (CPR; chest compression, shock, or medications to revive heart and breathing) if the heart or breathing stops.

An important question surfaces here: how do we know when we are at the end of life? This is answered by the attending physician, who after proper examination and deliberation, must come to the conclusion that the disease process is irreversible, incurable, and—in addition to that—will result in imminent demise.

What is imminent demise? Imminent may mean minutes, hours, days, or weeks. For medical purposes, if death will be within three to six months, the patient is considered terminal. Doctors can give artificial support in the form of breathing machines, dialysis, or nutrition to extend this process for more than six months. Since the interventions may be uncomfortable and yet not lead to recovery, the individual chooses a "natural death" via a DNR order.

There is an obvious problem with the idea of imminent demise. In many circumstances, doctors can tell quite clearly that death will occur soon. In others, doctors know that death is likely but can't say if it will be in three to six months. The problem becomes even more complicated in permanent coma.

The Illinois state website at illinois.gov provides a complete living will declaration. Here, we must deal with the next important concept, illustrated by the following excerpt:

> In the absence of my ability to give directions regarding the use of such death-delaying procedures, it is my intention that this declaration shall be honored by my family

and physician as the final expression of my legal right to refuse medical or surgical treatment and accept the consequences of such refusal.

This sentence is critical. First, one must declare that one is responsible for his or her decision. This takes the burden of decision making away from the family and relieves family members of any guilt or anguish. For this reason, it is so important to draw up a living will, or at the very least to discuss end-of-life desires. These desires trump the wishes of the family. As we shall see in the stories to follow, families may be emotional at this time and want to hang on and choose therapies that patients would never want. The living will declaration also overrides the health care power of attorney (HCPOA). The HCPOA is a document created by the patient when he or she is of sound mind and designates a person or persons to make decisions about health when the patient is unable to do so. A designee knows the health care values of the patient and will act in the best interests of the patient.

Why would a person want to draw up an advance directive? People see loved ones go through long illnesses at the end of life and are subsequently concerned about their own independence and dignity. Some never want to be in a nursing home while others don't want to suffer the painful effects of chemicals, tubes, needles, and bedsores at the end of life. Many don't want to rely on others to help them turn in bed or clean their bodies. They don't want to be fed into their stomachs if they can't eat by themselves. And many don't want to carry on if they lack the mental capacity to recognize their loved ones or to enjoy their environments. Individuals don't want the last stages of their lives remembered as prolonged illness.

Is a living will mandatory when you can't make health care decisions for yourself? No. Communicating your health care values clearly to a loved one, a friend, or a physician will suffice. This person should be available to speak for you. In a medical system, there is a hierarchy for substituted decision making: the spouse, adult children, parents, and siblings may speak on your behalf. Having said that, a written advance directive is always better.

In summary, a patient with a living will declares the following:

I relieve my family of all responsibilities and declare that A) if I am in a terminal condition and unable to make my health care decisions and/or B) if I am in a permanently unconscious state as determined by two physicians, then I direct my attending doctor as follows:

1. Do not do CPR, do not place me on life support, and do not provide me with artificial nutrition in any manner to extend my dying process.
2. Stop such treatment, including CPR, if such treatment has started.
3. Place a DNR Order in the chart.
4. Let me die naturally, take no action to postpone my death, providing me with only that care necessary to make me comfortable and to relieve my pain.

The wording above is similar that used by the states of Indiana, Illinois, and Ohio. Other states may interpret things differently, but a similar philosophy exists. Living wills in different states allow extended discussions on the type of comfort, nutrition, or hospital/hospice needs desired by a patient. Some states allow advance directives that detail a person's health care values.

It should be noted that living wills are often criticized because they can be vague. There is a concern that patients' choices may change over time. Patients are unable to make complex decisions even regarding current illnesses, so how are they expected to plan for an unknown future?

What is end of life? How do doctors know when that phase has been entered? The risk of death is always present once we are born! If we are born with certain problems, we may die in the first year of our lives. The body reaches peak tissue and strength at twenty-five to thirty years. After that time, the tissues no longer grow; they maintain themselves by replacement cells. The replacement cells in different tissues have diverse abilities to keep on replenishing. At some stage, the capacity to replenish goes away, and the body acquires more fat cells and scar tissue.

Vision is best around the age of twenty-five, and by age forty glasses are often needed to read. The hearing is sharpest around ten years of age; it declines even before we know it! At age fifty, we may only have 80 percent of the strength we had at age twenty-five. Whether we like it or not, the skin becomes wrinkled and bone structure changes. The brain, the heart, and the lungs all go through degenerative changes. In our middle fifties, the ability of deoxyribonucleic acid (DNA) to repair itself diminishes such that tissue damage and cancer risk become a problem. Most cultures around the world embrace this fact and that death is a natural part of life.

The average life span for an adult male in the United States is about seventy-eight years and is about eighty-one years for a female. This does not mean that an adult male will die around the age of seventy-eight; that just happens to be the average. As a matter of fact, if you are fifty years old and reading this, then you are one of those who is likely to live longer than the age of seventy-eight. All averages are a distribution on a bell-shaped curve (Figure 1). Some groups, as shown in the far-left columns on the graph, have a shorter life span (due to diseases, trauma, violence, and drugs, among other factors), while other groups, shown in the far right, live longer (due to factors like good genes and healthy living). Medicare.gov and some life insurance companies—such as Northwestern Mutual—put life span calculators on line. Life insurance companies calculate life span based on multiple factors.

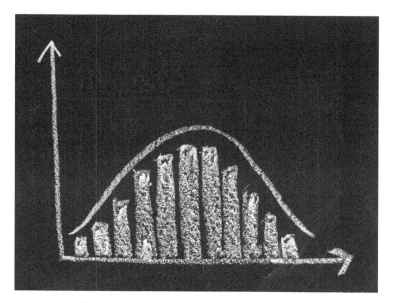

Figure 1: The bell-shaped curve is an important consideration in all the averages quoted in this book. (permission from fotosearch.com)

As we approach our genetic and physiologic life span, tissues are worn and their ability to sustain a cohesive body function declines. Life insurance companies decide our risk of death based on our diseases, lifestyle, work, income, education, and whether we smoke or drink, among other parameters. Diabetes, smoking, and high blood pressure affect the circulation of blood and diminish our ability to recover. (We will see this repeatedly in the stories that follow.) In the United States, we live stressful lives and/or lives of excess, yet we expect a long, healthy life. We are a young nation. Our age-defying philosophy, as it relates to death and dying, is what the drug companies and hospitals want us to embrace. Mostly, we see death as the enemy. The United States ranks twenty-sixth in life expectancy among developed nations, even though we spend the most money at the end of life.

Doctors know when critical organs have failed or are functioning very poorly even with optimal treatment. The symptoms, signs, and test results are often accurate for predicting organ failure such that life can no longer be sustained. In the chapters that follow, we will discuss organ failure and how doctors know the end may be near.

Two

The resuscitation

The cause of heart arrest is often an irregular rhythm of the pumping chambers (the ventricles) of the heart. The heart has two blood-receiving chambers (atria) and two ventricles. An integral coordinated rhythm keeps the heart circulating blood through the body, day and night. Muscles of the ventricles pump tirelessly and thus require a significant blood supply. The blood vessels of the heart—the coronary arteries—supply blood to these muscles.

As we age, the coronary arteries can get clogged with cholesterol plaques, calcium deposits, and blood clots, compromising circulation to the muscles (Figure 2). Lack of circulation through the coronary arteries can induce a chaotic rhythm of the ventricles. This chaotic rhythm (ventricular fibrillation) can result in loss of pumping of blood. (Even though it is a distinct phenomenon, think of a "Charlie horse" cramp in the legs, when you have been sitting in one spot for a long time and then you try to move, but nothing happens—just tingling and a cramp). Ventricular fibrillation causes circulation failure—a cardiac arrest.

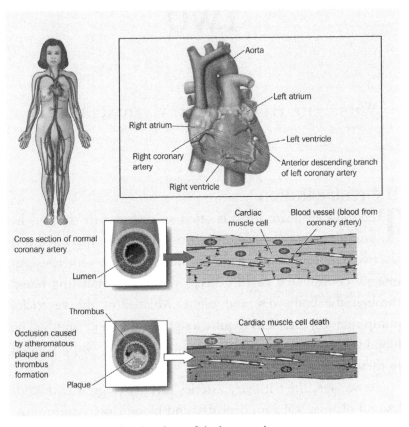

Figure 2: The chambers of the heart and coronary artery disease. (permission from fotosearch.com)

For medical students, residents, and young health care professionals, a cardiac arrest—or "code blue"—is an adrenaline rush. They want to participate in reviving or resuscitating a patient. The heartbeat has stopped or breathing has ceased, and the pulse is lost. Now it is up to the code team to get the patient back. The cardiopulmonary resuscitation (CPR) process requires teamwork, with a leader who directs the other members to perform certain tasks in hope of a positive outcome. The end result of successful CPR and advanced cardiac life support (ACLS) is recovery of the heart's normal rhythm. Delivery of an electric shock will often stop all chaotic rhythm and allow the natural rhythm to take over. The delivery of a quick shock is paramount, and thus it is monitored and documented to ensure the quality of CPR. If an electric shock is not immediately successful, the team will keep working. The team leader will monitor proper delivery of chest compressions. Compressions applied to the chest will result in blood flowing to the chest and, hopefully, into the arteries of the heart. An airway to the lungs is secured by the placement of a breathing tube. Respiratory therapists will use a bag to inflate lungs with air and then let them deflate. Medications such as adrenaline are injected, and blood tests are performed to monitor the progression of heart arrest. The heart rhythm is closely monitored, and resuscitation protocols are carried out accordingly.

How bad is a cardiac arrest?

Mrs. Sue Maynard Campbell's case was well publicized. She was full-time chair of the Association of Disabled Professionals and had served in the National Health System (NHS) Disabilities Rights Commission. The NHS is a governmental body that administers health care in the United Kingdom. Mrs. Maynard had a physical disability and was wheelchair dependent. In 1998, she presented to the hospital with a severe chest infection. A physician examined Mrs. Maynard and wrote "do not resuscitate" in her chart. He judged that if CPR was required, Mrs. Maynard's quality of life would be very poor due to her physical condition. The physician in question did not tell Mrs. Maynard that he was declaring her DNR. The doctor's decision did not go over very well with Mrs. Campbell. She was angry that someone had made a quality judgment about her life and its worth. In her case, if her lung infection became dangerous, being on a breathing machine would still likely bring about recovery and allow her to enjoy life at her previous functional level. Would she be denied this care just because she was wheelchair bound? She was appropriately angry about the whole situation and vowed never to go to a hospital again. Patients with disability fear they will be similarly labeled. The NHS has made efforts to quell these anxieties.

Why did her doctor think that the cardiac arrest would be too much for Mrs. Maynard?

A breathing tube inserted *before* the arrest would help Mrs. Maynard, so the DNR designation was an incorrect decision. However, had Mrs. Maynard gone into cardiac arrest with ongoing pneumonia, her recovery could have been problematic.

The success of CPR and advanced cardiac life support has little to do with being wheelchair bound but a lot to do with the patient's condition and the cause of cardiac arrest. Does the patient have heart or lung disease? Was there infection or pneumonia? Does the patient have massive blood loss? Does the patient have electrolyte problems? Was the oxygen level low before the heart arrest? Did blood clots in the lungs cause the arrest?

If CPR, including advanced cardiac life support is performed on a *hospitalized patient*, the likelihood that the individual will come out of heart arrest is about 60 percent. This means that for every-one hundred patients who go into arrest, sixty will have a recovered pulse. The other forty patients will die during the code. Out of the sixty who recover their pulse, forty will die during hospitalization. Only twenty will leave the hospital! And what shape will they be in at the time of discharge?

Out of hospital arrest patients are slightly different. If they receive proper CPR and early electric shock treatment (defibrillation), they have a good chance of doing well. Cities arrange their emergency services such that an ambulance can reach the location of a cardiac arrest victim quickly. If a victim has not been administered any CPR for about eight to ten minutes, the likelihood of recovery becomes very small. It is helpful if someone, such as a bystander, performs CPR. Patients who have a bystander perform CPR and who get an early return of rhythm have better survival odds than those who are found late in an arrest. Nonwitnessed arrests, patients who may have collapsed a long time before being found, don't do as well. Therefore, the chance for survival depends on where you live or who is with you. For instance, if you are in New York, the likelihood that an ambulance will reach you or that a bystander will administer CPR is lower than, for example, in Seattle, where emergency medical service is faster and bystander CPR more frequent. Therefore, everyone is encouraged to learn CPR and familiarize themselves with automated external defibrillators (AEDs).

Even so, out-of-hospital arrest patients can still die before reaching the hospital or soon after reaching a hospital. Of every-one hundred patients who have such out-of-hospital arrests, only ten to thirty may survive to be discharged from a hospital. Out of these ten to thirty patients who survive, many will have poor brain function; others will have some degree of physical limitation.

A nursing home patient suffering a heart arrest is unlikely to wake up and go back to his or her prearrest functional status. These patients commonly have advanced lung or heart disease, many are bedridden, or they have had small strokes. *Therefore, expecting a good outcome is not realistic and is the reason doctors recommend DNR for chronically ill patients.*

This brings us to the case of sixty-eight-year-old Brian. He had been ill for two days prior to presentation. A perforation of the bowel was diagnosed when he came to the emergency room. Surgeons had performed extensive surgery. Bowel content had soiled the abdominal cavity. At the end of surgery, there were multiple drains in his abdomen. Arriving at the intensive care unit from the operating room, Brian was unresponsive and on a ventilator. His blood pressure was low, and he was thus in need of the support of multiple medications called *vasopressors*. The practitioners and nurses were working diligently, correcting all the abnormalities they could.

Brian smoked and drank heavily, and he did not take care of his diabetes or high blood pressure. His blood vessels were narrowed and hardened with calcium deposits and cholesterol-like plaques. In medical terms, he had *peripheral vascular disease.*

It was no surprise under the circumstances that the circulation of blood was compromised. Many of Brian's fingers were turning blue as the medical team battled to control the shock.

The pressure repeatedly drifted down, requiring the administration of additional intravenous fluids (*fluid bolus*). As noted, Brian was on medication—vasopressors—that propped his blood pressure up; these had been titrated to maximum doses. To make matters worse, it appeared Brian had suffered a myocardial infarction (MI), or heart attack. An MI in Brian's condition would mean that the blood pressure was too low to send an adequate supply of blood through the coronary arteries. Heart muscles die as coronary circulation is increasingly compromised. Two hours after the surgery, Brian's heartbeat stopped and the code team rushed in to revive him. They pumped his chest and provided advanced cardiac life support, which recovered the pulse as well as the blood pressure.

Once the heart stops pumping blood, a stopwatch has been turned on. The brain is an organ that needs constant oxygen and blood flow. Loss of blood circulation means brain cells will start to die. The race is now on to reestablish circulation in the shortest amount of time possible. If the brain cells die or swell, the likelihood that the patient will remain in a permanent coma is relatively high. Loss of circulation affects other organs in addition to the brain, such as the kidneys. Such a patient is at risk for developing multiple organ problems. The problem is complicated because even after restoration of a pulse, the heart "wakes up" in the same problematic body conditions that caused the arrest in the first place. Brian's arrest was due to low blood pressure, MI, and acidity. All the ingredients were still ripe and present to make the heart stop again. CPR is not a treatment of disease; it is a temporary measure for reviving heartbeat, and it works in patients capable of sustaining it.

It is understood that CPR is an attempt and not a guaranteed success. If CPR continues for more than twenty-five or thirty minutes, health professionals know that the patient's chances of survival are dismal. At some stage, physicians must stop the process and pronounce the patient dead. Individuals do not understand these issues and continue to believe that CPR will bring everyone back to life; professionals understand the gravity of CPR and the fact that not everyone is a candidate for successful CPR.

In the United Kingdom, doctors will designate a patient DNR if the patient has made a declaration to that effect. Also, if a patient's condition is such that resuscitation is unlikely to succeed or if successful resuscitation would not be in patient's best interest because it would lead to poor quality of life, the doctor can declare the patient DNR after discussing it with the patient and or the patient's family.

In America, it is different. In Brian's case, things appeared to be progressing poorly. Again, that evening, a code blue was called, and again the code team rushed to the bedside. Once more, there was success in recovering a pulse. Brian's wife, Connie, could not take it anymore. She had to go home. She knew that the doctors were right. They had told her Brian would not make it, even with further CPR. They said it was futile and that CPR would just hurt Brian. Connie could not cope with that; he had to make it. The doctors had to keep going, no matter what.

Brian had uncontrolled accumulation of acids in his body (acidosis). When circulation to the tissues of the body is compromised, the cells do not receive enough oxygen to function. The energy metabolism in cells is skewed to produce large amounts of lactic acid. The lactic acid makes the blood extremely acidic. The organs of the body can't function, and the heart tends to stop. It is a terminal condition unless there is a way to improve circulation and lower the acid levels. Sometimes emergency dialysis is a temporary option, but with low blood pressure, this was not possible for Brian. Connie wanted Brian to have full support. She had said, "No matter what, keep him going." The doctors had done just that. But at some point in the care of a patient, the futility of care becomes clear to the providers.

Soon, the doctors asked Connie to come back to the hospital; it was a matter of short time. Connie came in and stood at the bedside staring at the monitor, the alarm going off periodically, the nurses working. She did not look at anyone or utter a single word. Her expectations from the system were shattered. The doctor stood by her side as Brian's heart rhythm slowed down and stopped. No CPR was performed. The doctors pronounced him deceased.

In the United States, the focus of care is based on patient autonomy (patients' wishes). If a patient desires a certain surgery, the doctors will offer it if it is feasible. The doctor will go over the pros and cons of a surgery, but will not offer it if the benefit is small or risk high. However, this standard often does not hold for CPR. It is presumed everybody would choose to receive it unless they have a DNR bracelet and a community DNR signed by family doctor prior to hospitalization. The use of CPR is expected for even the very ill, so their families are surprised when physicians ask whether they desire CPR.

Health-care providers are not obliged to do CPR if the patient has no scope of recovery, as in Brian's case. However, when families request it, physicians end up doing CPR three, four, or five times before there is ultimately no response to CPR. Hospitals and administrators are focused on family satisfaction, even if families insist on futile CPR.

Understandably Connie, as a spouse, was in shock and had a hard time coping. The staff tried to explain the issues, but failed to successfully comfort her. Consoling her was extremely difficult under the circumstances, as Connie could not emotionally process what the staff said. The emotional toll on staff members, too, is not to be underestimated. Young professionals, after intense effort, don't expect to fail the patient and the family; they take it hard. Not surprisingly, intensive care unit is stressful for the workers. To make a bad situation worse, estranged family members (usually children, some living out of town) demand full support in futile cases. There is no evaluation of these spokespersons. Do they truly speak for the patient and truly know the patient's desires? Do they have the necessary understanding of the issues to make a proper judgment? Do they have ulterior motives, or do unresolved emotions affect their decision making?

Three

A promise to keep

Human beings stop breathing at the end of their lives. That has been the case since the beginning—until, that is, innovative humans tackled polio.

Polio has been described for hundreds of years. In 1916, there was a massive outbreak in New York. Approximately twenty-seven thousand cases of polio were identified, resulting in six thousand deaths in the United States during that time.

The poliovirus has a predilection for neurons, particularly those in the spinal cord. Leg weakness and loss of muscle strength are common problems in affected patients. Young patients develop palsy or weakness and are often left with a lifelong limp or undeveloped muscles. The virus can start to affect higher regions of the spinal cord, all the way up to the brain stem. At this stage, it is called *bulbar polio.* When the brain stem is affected, patients may lose the ability to cough and breathe, so they can die from breathing difficulties. This was the primary cause of polio deaths in the early 1900s. The mortality rate for patients with bulbar polio was as high as 90 percent.

With thousands of patients affected and dying, there had to be a way to keep patients breathing. The 1920s saw an emergence of iron lungs. The patient is placed in a cylinder, which can create a vacuum. The vacuum allows the chest to rise outward, allowing air to move into the chest cavity, thus causing the patient to inhale. In the next cycle, the pressure in the iron lung chamber returns and pushes the chest inward, causing the patient to exhale. Iron lungs were useful in helping hundreds of patients. Many patients spent decades of their lives supported by these devices. There are, however, some limitations to the concept of the iron lung. The throat and upper lungs must be clear of secretions and be patent, or open. With bulbar polio, this ability is gone. It is also difficult to take care of a patient in such a contraption.

In the early 1900s, the surgical procedure tracheotomy became more prevalent (Figure 3). Tracheostomy tube placement allowed access to the windpipe, thus bypassing the airway and secretion issues. (A tracheostomy is the hole in the neck; a tracheotomy is the surgical procedure to create it). Small rubber bellows pump air into the lungs through this tracheostomy tube. During the polio epidemics of the early 1950s, hundreds of volunteers, students, and nurses compressed airbags (bellows) to provide air to patients with polio.

During those few decades, half a million people died of polio. Throughout the peak period of the Copenhagen epidemic, there were an estimated three hundred patients with tracheostomies and thousands of volunteers taking turns to keep their wards alive. Positive-pressure ventilators were already available, but were refined over the coming years. These are mechanized bellows that push air into the lungs through a breathing tube or the tracheostomy tube.

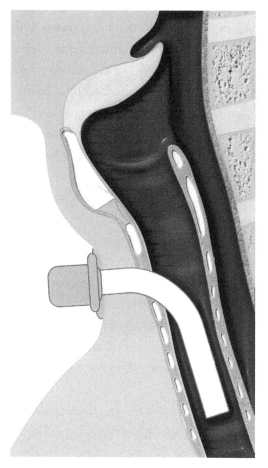

Figure 3: Cross section of windpipe. Surgically placed tracheostomy tube is standard for long-term ventilator care. (permission from fotosearch.com)

Providing prolonged care to patients attached to sophisticated devices takes specialized units. Modern intensive care units can support heart, lung, kidney, brain, blood, and bowel functions, as well as provide facilities for complex surgeries and care of massive trauma, massive burn, and complex transplant patients.

At age sixty-two, Nora had been diagnosed with progressive muscle weakness due to amyotrophic lateral sclerosis (ALS), or Lou Gehrig's disease. She could not walk very much and now had a hard time getting out of bed. While eating, she started dropping things from her hands. More recently, she coughed while eating as if the food were going down the windpipe.

Several days before presentation, Nora was finding it difficult to catch her breath so she came to the hospital. When the doctors examined her, Nora's oxygen level was slightly low, but her carbon dioxide level was high. Carbon dioxide removal is an important function of the lungs. The reduction in capacity to take a deep breath will often result in accumulation of carbon dioxide. ALS is caused by loss of the motor neurons, which control muscle activity. ALS ultimately affect breathing muscles. The ability to cough decreases over time. As the cough mechanism becomes weak, the secretions tend to stay at the dependent parts of the lungs. Nora's chest x-ray was suggestive of plugs in the bottom parts of the lungs.

Nora's son Frank manufactured cabinets and ran a successful business. He knew about his mother's condition from all the previous discussions with the doctors and specialty center visits. The family knew the disease was progressive and that death was likely within a period of a few years. Nora had been introduced to the concept of hospice; however, neither she nor her son were ready yet. Frank had convinced Nora that he was going to take care of her at home, no matter what, and would never put her in a nursing home. Frank had read about this disease, looked into cough-assist and bi-level positive airway pressure (BiPAP) devices, and was prepared to have a ventilator at home if needed. BiPAP is a snugly fitting mask that provides inhalation assistance.

During this hospitalization, the secretion buildup was significant, and Nora was developing pneumonia. Her carbon dioxide level was too high, but BiPAP—often helpful with the movement of air—was not right for Nora due to the secretions. Her doctors discussed the options, including the breathing machine and subsequent tracheotomy. She understood the concept of the home ventilator, and that is what she wanted. Even when patients choose the home ventilator, they can ask for home hospice support. In that case, the hospice team will provide supplemental care at home. Usually, though, it means that if a patient deteriorates, the focus will be on comfort care.

But that was not what the son wanted. The son wanted Nora to continue to live as long as possible on the ventilator. "Full code" meant that if her condition became critical, Nora's son wanted her back in the hospital for treatment—aggressive treatment including CPR if needed. The patient was in agreement with her son.

After being on the breathing machine for a few days, Nora underwent a tracheotomy and a feeding tube placement, and was discharged to a long-term acute care hospital (LTACH/long-term hospital). The idea was that the family would learn about ventilators from the long-term hospital. Home arrangement for a ventilator include oxygen, suction, and a specialized bed. The family is trained in alarms, suctioning, providing skin care, and assisting the patient with daily care.

Unfortunately, Nora's course of treatment was complicated by an ileus, or bowel slowing. Her stomach did not tolerate feeding. Providers diagnosed Nora with *clostridium difficile colitis*, a bacterial overgrowth in the colon that is a common problem for patients on long-term antibiotics. Frequent watery bowel movements and distension were causing discomfort. The problem was significant enough that Nora required full intravenous nutrition, called *total parenteral nutrition* (TPN), for almost two weeks.

After a month in the long-term hospital, Nora was still not quite ready for home. The family partly trained on the breathing machine for home and learned how to suction and keep the catheters clean. They were educated on turning, changing, and tube feeding.

After almost two months at the long-term hospital, Nora was discharged home. The son and his wife took care of her. Many families provide great care to ventilator-dependent patients at home. It is an arduous task and success depends on the mind-set of the caregivers. The level of care depends on the individual patient and his or her disease burden. For the family, this is a life-changing event. The support effort requires total dedication by one or more family members. Alarms on Nora's machine went off periodically at night as she needed clearing of secretions with suction. The family had a visiting nurse for several hours a day who provided basic care. When the visiting nurse was not there, changing Nora's diaper three to four times a day was exhausting.

Caregiver fatigue was setting in after a few weeks. Nora had become completely bedridden and had lost all her muscle mass. She was often teary eyed, but smiled at her family. One day, the alarm kept beeping despite frequent suctioning. The family was scared when Nora bled through the tracheotomy tube. The visiting nurse recommended transfer back to the hospital. This time, Nora was treated for infection of the lungs. Eventually, though, patient and family were more open to home hospice. The focus shifted to comfort.

There are many cases of years of excellent care given to ventilator patients at home. Unfortunately, most patients encounter pneumonia over time, as well as urine or stomach problems. The human body is not meant for lying in bed for any length of time. In this particular case, the patient did not have any specific advance directives and was able to participate in decision making throughout her care. Nora and her family knew that the prognosis was poor, but she tried to forge on since many patients do live longer. Advanced ALS is truly a terminal condition, and we have to accept it as such. However, acceptance is a challenge for many, and the care becomes a road of discovery through hurdles. It is a physical, emotional, and financial fight. Ultimately, death and the dying experience are dependent on the spiritual and cultural fiber of patients and their families.

If nobody accepted death as natural, imagine how many patients would be on life support in nursing homes? In the age of advanced technology and artificial prolongation of death, tremendous confusion is generated when decisions are left to loved ones who don't know what it all means.

Four

I Am Ready

Individual health preferences

Naru is a small, quiet man. He has suffered three strokes so far. During his first stroke, he had right-sided weakness. After being in bed for a day or two, he started therapy. The first phase was sitting upright in bed, feet dangling to the side. He would lean quite a bit, almost to the point of tipping back into the bed; the therapist would support him upright. Over time, Naru was able to pivot to the chair. His right hand gained strength rapidly, but the right leg remained weak. Nevertheless, Naru was determined to walk: first with a walker, then with a cane, and then independently.

Naru could smile with half of his face; the right half was paralyzed. This was a shame because Naru had a perfectly calm, Zen-like smile before. Saliva now seeped out when he opened his mouth. Naru worked hard with a speech therapist and gradually began expressing a few words. Initially, only jumbled words came out; later, he could say his name. The ability to speak a sentence took months of trying to read kindergarten books aloud. Naru had great difficulty remembering the names of members of his family. Later, Naru said that immediately after his stroke, he could not formulate thoughts in his mind, nor could he express them.

A few years after his initial stroke, Naru wanted to drive. He was seventy-two and said he had recovered from the attack. He was prepared, but his family was not. The inability to drive would prove to be devastating for him. But that is the same challenge that families face all over the country. Inability to drive means dependence on somebody else. In his family's eyes, Naru did not have the necessary faculties to drive; they thought he would hurt himself and possibly others. It took a fair amount of convincing Naru to let go of the idea of driving since he is fiercely independent.

People in Naru's circumstances have coordination and balance issues, as well as weak eyesight, but some are determined to drive. Reportedly, younger people aged eighteen to twenty-nine years are involved in more car accidents than people aged sixty-five years or older, mainly because the elderly drive less. Most importantly, if there is an accident involving an older individual, the likelihood of death is high.

That was almost eight years ago. Since then, Naru has probably had at least two more strokes. He follows the activities of his grandkids and tends a little garden. News on TV and the computer are of keen interest, but take great effort to decipher. Naru has said many times that he is "ready." At age eighty, he has lived a fruitful life and doesn't have any other desires. He has also been known to say, "Just shoot me the day I can't get out of bed." In the meantime, he has made a living will expressing that he wouldn't want life-support in the case of critical illness. In reality, had he not created a living will, it would have been fine. Naru had already expressed his desire, which the family could convey to physicians. He had said, "Shoot me if I cannot get out of bed."

With that background, what does a statement like that mean? *How do the doctors interpret it?*

An inability to get out of bed is not a terminal condition. A hip fracture could make Naru unable to get out of bed. But it was clear that he did not want to live dependent on others. He is a proud man.

So, if Naru came to the hospital with a new stroke, couldn't get out of bed, and needed a breathing machine, then what should the doctors do? Should the doctors put him on life support for respiratory failure? Or does his living will take effect? Should the doctors keep him comfortable?

In this hypothetical situation, Naru has not the met the living will criteria. Since the physicians cannot determine the terminal condition or permanence of coma right away, they would provide aggressive support until they could determine it. But more importantly, is that what Naru would want?

When asked about this, Naru thought it over and said, "If I can come back to my current level of function, you can support me." In his mind, the second two strokes were relatively minor and had not left him with new problems. When asked, "How would the doctor know if the function is going to come back unless they put you on life support, at least for a few days, and observed you?" A big stroke causing respiratory failure would likely cause new deficits and a bedridden state, at least for some time. Naru would be in a dependent situation during the time of recovery. Finally, he said, "After such a big stroke, I would not be the same. If a stroke is severe enough to cause respiratory failure, I don't want life support; just keep me comfortable."

Separate from the living will is an ability to choose the level of care at the time of admission to the hospital. (Figure 4). The attending physician signs the level of care request form after he or she understands the desires of the patient regarding choices of life support or CPR. Naru or his family would, upon admission, indicate that he wanted DNR status. This form is easy to complete in the hospital and requires no attorney or fee. Patients' desires to be designated DNR should be made known to the family and documented in the chart by the provider.

Living Will	Patient creates a document directing the care at end of life. It is a formal document made available when needed. Scope is narrow and related to terminal state.
Health Care Power of Attorney	Patient designates person(s) to direct health care when patient can't. It is a formal document to be made available when needed. Scope is broad and is good for any medical condition.

Do Not Resuscitate (DNR)/Level of Care	May not require patient to sign any forms. It can be verbal instructions to providers regarding care in event of arrest. Scope is limited to CPR or comfort in a facility.
Community DNR	Patient or guardian sign this form with help of a physician. It is to be produced by the family in case of emergency. Often a DNR bracelet is worn by the patient. Community DNR tells the medical system that CPR is not desired. Scope is limited to CPR but effective everywhere.
Expressed wishes	Patient conveys wishes regarding care to the family who speaks on patient's behalf when needed. Scope is broad but less formal. If the next of kin is not the spouse then agreement among all children or siblings is required in some circumstances.

Figure 4: Options commonly used (simplified here)
when patient is unable to make decisions.

A "hospital DNR" is good for one admission and needs to be revisited. DNR status can be broken down into different components of resuscitation. If your heart were to stop, would you want electric shock (cardioversion) to try to revive the rhythm? Should the providers inject medications into your veins to attempt to restore your rhythm? Would you want staff to perform CPR to try to revive the heartbeat? Would you want to have a breathing tube inserted to breathe for you (intubation) if you were to stop breathing?

DNR discussions require some thought. A health care provider should assist in answering questions as to the goals of care and the best choices. In a circumstance where a patient has a limited life expectancy but has a possibility of a brief irregular heart rhythm, it may be acceptable to choose cardiac shock without intubation. On the other hand, a patient with advanced emphysema (a lung disease) may be willing to be placed on a ventilator for a few days. He or she may choose not to have heart shocks or chest compressions in case of cardiac arrest and just want nature to take its course. The goals of care should be at the heart of these decisions.

Naru's case is not unique. Naru had some disability, but he was not willing to have any further disability. Even if the next stroke does not result in respiratory failure, it may result in a degree of disability that is undesirable. A government census suggests 56.7 million people—18.7 percent of the population, or almost one in five people—live with some degree of disability. The disability may be a communication, mental, or physical problem. The point is that disability can affect the perception of quality of health and enjoyment of life such that it makes a person review their desires regarding aggressive care. Disability should not be equated with lack of enjoyment. Disability also does not mean a person is unhealthy.

Is there a way to grade Naru's function and disability?

The Barthel scale is a simple function-measurement scale. The Barthel scale grades mobility, grooming, and other activities of daily living (ADL). Ten tasks are scored. When the total score is one hundred, one is fully functional; when it is less than twenty-five, the person is extremely dependent. If the Barthel score is forty, one may be in a situation where there is need of assistance with food, may have bowel accidents, or may require substantial use of a wheelchair. Due to its simplicity, the scale allows providers to monitor decline or progress quickly. It does not, however, consider mental abilities and quality of life.

Naru used an online Barthel calculator. He scored ninety, needing some help with grooming occasionally and with stairs. In reality, his functional capacity was not too bad. But Naru wanted much more out of himself. He wanted to drive and travel independently! He wanted to understand writing (without putting in a huge effort) and, most importantly, he wanted to write. But, Naru could see that a score of sixty would be too much dependence for his liking. If he had another big stroke and his ADL were reduced to less than sixty on the Barthel scale, he hoped that he would just go in peace. If he were incapable of eating, he would not want artificial feeding. Maybe that would be the cause of his demise. Or, if his doctors told him he had less than six months to live, he would just seek hospice help. The nursing home was not a favorite option, but having family take care of him was even lower on the list.

It should be noted that a person who has experienced new deficits will adjust over time and will view his or her situation in more acceptable terms. He or she may find joy and happiness in lesser-functioning state. Therefore, priorities should be made very clear.

This chapter highlights what next of kin must convey to doctors. What were patient's true wishes? It is understood that the family's true wish may be to keep on holding on to the patient. Making a patient live in less than their desired state would be wrong. Similarly, artificially pushing death back may have no advantage for the one suffering, even when he or she has expressed the wish that everything possible be done to prolong life.

Section 2

CATASTROPHIC ILLNESS

Five

Prognostications in an intensive care unit

Abby turned seventy-six, and to celebrate her birthday, her daughter and granddaughter had made a cake. Her son's family lived out of town. Abby had diabetes and high blood pressure that were well controlled by her medications. Retired and widowed, she now lived with her pet dog. She returned home one day, slipped, and fell in the garage. She hit her head and passed out. Her neighbors found her on the floor of the garage. When the medics brought her to the hospital, she did not respond to doctors calling her name. Both her pupils reacted to light. When the nurse pinched her arms, she stretched them out, extending them to the side in a response called *extensor response.* Health professionals calculated her coma scale score. This scale gives health professionals an idea of the severity of the coma, and it can help predict patient outcomes.

The human skull is a solid box. The brain is a soft tissue within this box. Different linings, or *meninges,* support the tissues of the brain inside the skull. The brain jiggles upon a sudden movement of the head. The meninges support the brain tissue during that moment. There are certain points at which the meninges anchor the brain to the skull. Here, the soft tissue of the brain is held tight to the inner parts of the skull. The meninges also allow blood vessels to pass into the tissues of the brain.

With a sudden movement of the brain, such as that caused by a rapid acceleration or deceleration, the brain tissues will lag behind the actual skull (like gelatin in a moving plate) and strain against the meninges. The tissues of the brain can bruise, tear, or develop contusions at these anchoring points or farther down. Blood can collect from a tear of the vessels within different meninges.

Abby underwent a quick evaluation in the emergency room. No other injuries were found other than a bruise on the head. A brain computer tomography (CT) scan suggested there was a small amount of blood collecting between the meninges and some blood within the tissues of the brain. There was a subtle change at the junction of the white matter and gray matter. The gray matter tissue of the brain has a different density than the underlying white matter. A head injury from a fall can result in differential shearing movements of these two types of brain tissue. Many neurons are long cells that traverse from the outer gray matter of the brain all the way down to the spine. Some brain cells may swell and die because of a sudden pull and tear along the length, as shown in Figure 5. This tearing and shearing injury of the neurons is called *diffuse axonal injury.* Diffuse axonal injury may have long-term consequences for recovery.

The swelling of the brain and blood within the brain can cause increased pressure in the skull cavity. There can only be a limited amount of gelatin in the container; the addition of fluid and blood to the skull cavity (cranial cavity) will result in high pressures. High pressures on brain tissues may prevent the brain from functioning. At extremely high pressure, blood will stop flowing into the skull or the brain tissue will start to extrude through skull openings—a condition called herniation. Of course, fragments of the skull bone can penetrate the tissues of the brain.

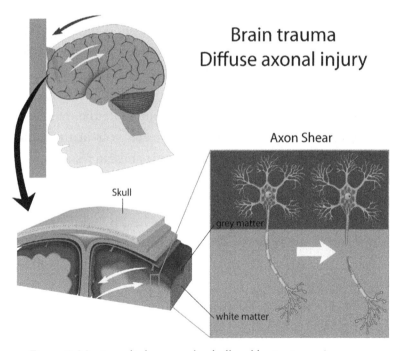

Figure 5: Meninges lie between the skull and brain tissue. A trauma can result in bleeding within the meninges and within the brain tissue. The inset shows gray and white matter, diffuse axonal injury as a tear of the axon. (permission from fotosearch.com)

Abby's fall seemed minor. Why did she not wake up right away? If a roofer weighing two hundred twenty pounds falls from about thirty feet, when he hits the ground he is falling at a rate of about thirty miles per hour (mph). It takes about 1.43 seconds to hit the ground. It would have an effect equal to 3300 pounds of weight falling from three feet. The body comes to a full stop from a speed of thirty mph almost instantly; that amount of energy at impact is tremendous. If the fall is on the head, the forces are deadly. All body parts, soft or hard, can be gravely injured, torn, broken, or crushed.

A simple fall can result in bleeding around the brain tissue or between the meninges. A seemingly small blow on the head can cause a concussion. A concussion is a shaken brain, causing confusion or black out. A brief concussion is a common type of traumatic brain injury (TBI) and represents the majority of more than a million TBIs that occur each year in the United States. Even mild TBI can be problematic and can result in weeks of irritability, headache, loss of concentration, muscle stiffness, dizziness, and inability to sleep, among other problems. Sports are a constant source of concern. In a healthy adult, recovery commonly occurs in a few weeks. In people who abuse alcohol or have dementia, TBI may be difficult to diagnose and may require careful investigation.

TBI causing loss of alertness or blackout for six hours can be considered moderate, while loss of consciousness longer than six hours is considered severe. Moderate to severe TBI can cause long-term effects. There is an association with increased risk for seizures, Parkinson's brain diseases, and possibly dementia. Long-term and permanent loss of function, such as inability to walk, inability to learn, and memory loss are possible.

Abby needed the support of an intensive care unit. Nurses placed a tube down her nose into her stomach. They watched her breathing carefully and wanted to make sure her pulse and her blood pressure remained stable. In fact, her blood pressure was low, requiring additional fluids. She had an oxygen mask on her face. Abby remained in a poor state of responsiveness, but her breathing performed well enough on its own. Abby periodically, had phlegm in the back of her throat, which the nurses suctioned clear.

Her daughter Molly and granddaughter Debbie were at the bedside, apparently worried and tearful. Abby's son David was on his way from Texas. Doctors had told them that Abby had a significant injury. A magnetic resonance imaging (MRI) scan of the head suggested swelling of the brain, white matter changes, and a small amount of blood within the brain tissues; however, no surgery was planned. An intracranial pressure measurement would possibly be required on suspicion of increasing pressures. CT scans can be helpful in making decisions for care and in predicting the outcome. A normal CT scan does not mean everything will be fine. Given the patient's condition and type of head trauma, one in ten with a normal CT scan may still die. Also, a CT scan may change over time. Careful examination of the patient is still an important part of providing a prognosis.

On the fourth day of hospitalization, Abby displayed some eye opening; she also squirmed around, but did not look at the staff or family members. Periodically, she wiggled with agitation and started breathing fast. If her eyelids were forced open, her eyes roved from one side to the other, but did not focus. She was feverish and had a lot more secretions in her lungs now. A number of patients with significant brain injury end up on breathing machines soon after presentation. Abby had escaped that so far.

She might still need a breathing machine to recover. David agreed to life support. *But what was her outlook?*

Doctors talk about survival and recovery based on their experience. Trauma surgeons will predict good or bad outcomes based on their examination and the overall picture. Large databases allow research teams to predict and calculate the outcome. One such database is published by the International Mission for Prognosis and Analysis of Clinical Trials in TBI (IMPACT). IMPACT investigators have created a calculator. The investigators take many studies representing thousands of patients and come up with a way of telling if the outcome will be good or bad. The calculator analyzes the likelihood of death. This particular calculator is published on the Internet at TBI-impact.org; it requires information on the patient's age, physical examination, CT scan, and other lab tests.

The calculator assessed the probability of Abby's death at 67 percent; it also assessed at 91 percent the probability of a poor outcome at six months. A poor outcome means a significantly dependent condition—often, a bedridden state in a nursing home. Even for patients who do okay after such an injury, there is an increased chance of seizures, memory loss, or Alzheimer's disease. But even without the specific calculations, the trauma doctors predicted a poor recovery.

It should be noted that studies show a majority of families doubt a doctor's ability to predict outcome, particularly bad outcomes.

David felt that his mom would want all possible interventions; however, given the poor outlook, Molly was not so sure. Abby's secretions improved with antibiotics. She did not need the breathing tube. Nutrition, however, was an issue. She was either too sleepy or too agitated. There was no way she was going to swallow food. The only option was to place a feeding tube right into the stomach through a small surgery, with the help of a scope. The procedure is called a *percutaneous endoscopic gastrostomy* (PEG). The temporary feeding tube normally placed down the nose can stay in place for a few weeks but would not allow for discharge from the hospital. After a few days, nose injury, sinus infections, and general care of the patient become issues. Since the family wanted to have some time to monitor Abby's progress, they agreed to the placement of the feeding tube. PEG was carried out on the tenth day of Abby's hospitalization.

On the twelfth day, she was transferred to the nursing home. At the nursing home, Abby still had problems with coughing and completely clearing her secretions. Her alertness remained low. Molly visited every evening, but she could not get any focused attention from her mom.

Abby returned to the hospital two weeks later with a serious case of recurrent pneumonia. A CT scan of her chest not only suggested pneumonia but a large blood clot in her lungs. Clotting of blood in the legs is also a big problem for hospitalized patients. Hospitals have protocols for preventing this problem. A clot in the leg can dislodge and settle in the lungs. This may cause very low oxygen levels. Emergency room doctors wanted to place a breathing tube to support Abby. Molly didn't want this; she talked to David over the phone. Abby was documented as DNR. The family wanted the further course to be natural and to only provide comfort at this stage. Abby died two days later.

In this case, there was no advance directive. The patient had not spoken to the family about her end-of-life wishes. She had a sudden event that took her from healthy function to a life-threatening situation. She was unable to express her wishes, and the children had to make decisions for her. The children were intelligent and level-headed; they asked appropriate questions. The doctors discussed the progress and options at each turn of her illness. Ultimately, the patient was designated DNR.

What if Abby was an 18-year-old? In an 18-year-old patient with similar injuries, of course, doctors would continue to offer care. Many of these young patients do slowly improve. Most need months of rehabilitation. Once recovery starts, they must go through a phase of assimilation into their world. Learning disability, limited concentration, communication gaps, and physical limitations may leave such patients developmentally behind other same-age youths. The brain has particular plasticity in the young, so many do make progress.

Problems related to level of care or how much to do don't come up as frequently when treating the young. It is taken for granted that all efforts will be made unless providing such efforts will be of no use. IMPACT calculator would predict better mortality and outcome results for the young given similar conditions.

Six

The Confused Brain: Delirium

Reliving an experience

Alertness and interaction are critical to humans. Imagine bringing your loved one to the hospital in an interactive and quite alert state. The next day, you walk in and the person is difficult to rouse. In addition, your loved one is tied down with restraints in a bed. To make the matter worse, the person is periodically shouting, angry, and fighting the restraints. It is very distressing. What happened?

For a health care professional, this is a daily issue. The fact remains that confusion is very common in hospitalized patients and much more so in an intensive care unit setting. Half of older patients with hip fractures may get confused about their whereabouts and the time, and become agitated. When patients see things that are not there—for example, spiders on the wall or a cat in the closet—they are hallucinating. The combination of confusion and agitation or sleepiness is called *delirium*. Hallucination is common in delirium. Delirium can affect

47

healthy young brains, but it is more common in patients with advanced age, patients with early dementia, and patients on multiple medications—particularly pain medications.

Health-care professionals ask simple orientation questions like the following regarding time, place, and person: What time is it? What year is it? Where are you? Are you at home? What's your name? Do you remember my name?

To patients, these questions are irritating. However, this is a way to identify problems early. If a person with chronic alcohol use wakes up from a surgery and then receives a shot of morphine, the time and place are difficult to figure out. Very quickly, the mind wanders. What has happened? What is this place? Who are these people? Very soon, there is bewilderment; anger; and, often, hallucination. What are those spiders doing on the wall? I must get out of here now. Let me out of here! Often, such a person is given Valium-type medications to calm him or her down. He or she will likely go to sleep, but wake up again in an even worse state of bewilderment. The patient's brain uses clues to figure out where the he or she might be, what time it might be, and who might be at the bedside or in the room. These tasks are performed based on memory, logic, and orientation cues. A dark room in the middle of the day, pain medications, abnormal electrolytes, low oxygen, alcohol use, early dementia, and a tied-down state, among other things, will make it less possible for a patient to get the cues lined up—which brings us to the story at hand.

Alan was on a newly developed blood thinner for irregular heart rhythm. Irregular heartbeat predisposes a patient to clots forming in the heart due to stagnated blood. Clots can be dangerous as they may travel from the heart and lodge in many places, including the brain. Alan was on a new blood thinner to prevent clot formation in the heart. Some of the newer blood thinners are easy to use as they don't require frequent blood testing. Unfortunately, many of these blood thinners don't have a "reversal" option. Reversal is required in some cases of bleeding, particularly in critical areas like the brain. In such cases, you want blood to clot quickly. You want to rapidly reverse the effects of the blood thinner.

At the age of ninety, Alan was active. One morning he went to pick up the paper and slipped. He fell, but stood up; his wife noticed a small bruise on his head. He was a stoic old man and denied that he had any pain in his hip or arm, but later complained of a headache. Subsequently that day, he felt weak on the right side. He then started to have seizures. Alan never actually woke up very well after the seizures. The CT scan of his head was suggestive of blood collecting in the meninges of the brain (Figure 6).

Alan was confused in the hospital and kept on pulling at the lines and tubes attached to him, wanting to get up and out of the bed. The nurses had no choice but to tie his hands or else he might hurt himself. Alan got wilder by the minute; not understanding restraints made him angry. His nurse wanted to administer a sedative or a calming medication called Ativan. This Valium-group drug also induces sleep and suppresses anxiety, but may prolong confusion. Another calming group is the antipsychotic medication group, which may work well for delirium; however, in Alan's case, antipsychotics could cause seizures. All medications have one problem or another, none being foolproof. Careful monitoring of brain function dictates the need for further testing or the urgency of surgery, and there was concern that such medications could interfere with this evaluation.

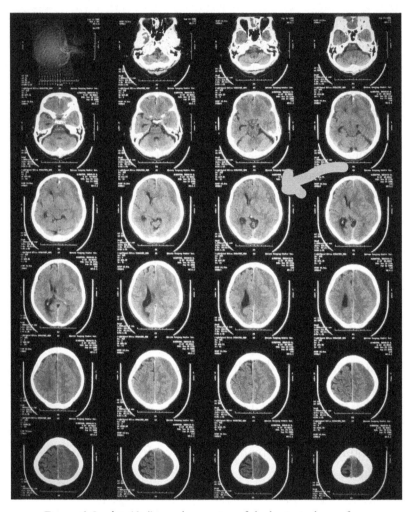

Figure 6: In this (6x4) panel, a section of the brain is shown from the bottom of the skull to top of the skull. This panel of scans focuses on the tissue of the brain and meninges. Several slices show blood collecting within the skull and shifting the brain. The arrow depicts this shift. (permission from fotosearch.com)

The blood collecting around Alan's brain is called a *subdural hematoma*. The surgeon explained that the blood could be drained and that it might help save his life, but she was not sure if the bleeding tendency caused by the blood thinner had completely resolved. She couldn't guarantee that the blood wouldn't ooze back into that area. She was also worried that, given the patient's advanced age, he might have prolonged confusion. However, the physicians felt that death would occur without intervention.

The Centers for Disease Control and Prevention (CDC) posted the following report on their home and recreation safety website:

> One out of five falls causes a serious injury such as broken bones or a head injury. Each year, 2.5 million older people are treated in emergency departments and 700,000 patients a year are hospitalized because of a fall injury, most often because of a head injury or hip fracture. Adjusted for inflation, the direct medical costs for fall injuries are $34 billion annually. People above age 65 constitute about 13% of our country's population but account for 40% of hospitalization with an average of 5.6 days spent in a hospital.

Alan's case exemplifies this report. Long-term recovery is a challenge after such falls. This age group already has weaker muscles and may have chronic conditions like high blood pressure, diabetes mellitus, and emphysema. Bed rest and reduced activity for even a few days can weaken them dramatically. Bone density is low in this population, with doctors asking patients to take calcium and vitamin D supplements. Bone-building medications may also be helpful. Engaging in regular exercise, including lifting small weights, is recommended. Doing so will reduce some of the injuries.

But Alan's case went a step further. Confusion and delirium affect 14 to 56 percent of hospitalized elderly and result in long-term neurological issues, such as memory problems, depression, and disorientation. Delirium adds several percentage points to the probability of death and a poor outcome. For example, the probability of mortality with a TBI–impact score of 80 percent will look much worse in patients who have prolonged delirium.

Dora, Alan's wife of six decades, was at the bedside as much as she could be. She had her hair in a neat bun. She was holding his hand with small frail hands as she related his problems from two years before. Alan had developed a kidney stone requiring hospitalization and experienced prolonged confusion during that time. For a few days, he was not himself. She recalled that he had never wanted to live like that for even a day and was now distressed by his current state.

For elderly patients with mild dementia or with periodic confusion, home is the safest place. It provides a familiar tether to which the mind can attach and stay oriented. Hospitalized patients lose that tether. Unfortunately for hospitalized patients, it is a catch-22 situation: they are not home, so they are confused; they are confused, so doctors won't let them go home. Many patients after hip surgery or other smaller procedures go to a nursing home for therapy. They are often given light pain medications, and they suddenly become disoriented for days and are unable to recover.

Dora did not want any surgeries for her husband; she asked instead for hospice care. Hospice services would help set up everything she needed for home to allow Alan to spend the rest of his days there; he would want it that way. The hospice caregivers would oversee his comfort and pain.

It should be noted that there is a worry that *early* designation of DNR will be a "self-fulfilling prophecy." Doctors decide that the outcome will be bad, designate the patient DNR, and do not provide what could be lifesaving care, resulting in patient death. This will reaffirm the doctor's prophecy that the patient will have poor outcome.

In this case, there was no advance directive, but the patient had lived through an experience of delirium that helped his wife decide against aggressive care.

Seven

Multiorgan Failure

How aggressive care is provided

Bill was a construction worker. At the age of 61, he was also a heavy smoker. His medical problems began with pain in the legs while walking. After dealing with it for months, he finally saw a doctor; she was concerned about circulation of blood and ordered an ultrasound of the blood vessels of his abdomen and legs. Ultrasound revealed an aneurysm of Bill's aorta. The aorta is a large blood vessel (artery) that carries the blood from the heart down to other organs of the abdomen and to the legs. The blood pressure in the aorta is high. An aneurysm is an abnormal weakness of the aorta wall leading to deformation; it can rupture and suddenly bleed massive amounts of blood into the abdominal cavity, resulting in sudden death. (Figure 7). An aneurysm can progress without many symptoms. Hospitals offer ultrasound screening to identify aneurysms in high-risk patients.

Upon obtaining information from the ultrasound, his doctor placed Bill on blood pressure medications and arranged an appointment with a surgeon to repair that aneurysm.

Normal

Abdominal Aortic Aneurysm

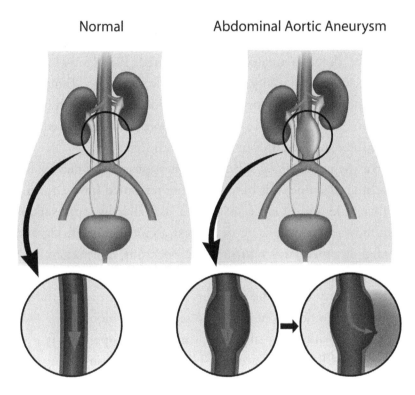

Figure 7: Abdominal aorta and aneurysm rupture.
(permission from fotosearch.com)

Bill had a strong personality with a booming voice, and he would do only what he wanted. His wife Diane was quiet and meek. The daughter Liz who was 18, was the only one who could convince Bill to do anything.

As it happened, Bill woke up with some back pain and later collapsed at work. This was not noticed immediately by Bill's co-workers, and it was not very clear how long he was down. Bill was pale and barely breathing when they discovered him. Paramedics rushed him to the emergency room. He was in shock; his blood pressure was extremely low. An urgent CT scan of his abdomen suggested that the aneurysm had ruptured. Blood was leaking into his abdominal cavity. Very soon, he was on a breathing machine and into an operating room. His body was pumped full of fluids and blood. Surgeons repaired his aorta and transferred him to the intensive care unit in critical condition.

For the next two days, Bill was unresponsive and needed the breathing machine. His blood pressure remained low, requiring further fluid and blood transfusions, as well as vasopressors. A complication occurred: he developed a clot in his left leg and needed an emergency return to the operating table. Even after the evacuation of the clot, part of his leg below the left ankle remained very blue. The surgeons thought that part of the leg might need to be amputated because of loss of blood flow.

On the third day after the surgery, Bill opened his eyes but did not follow commands. His exam was concerning and prompted the ordering of a CT scan of his head. The CT scan revealed a stroke affecting the left side of his brain.

Bill's recovery was a struggle. By the eighth day, he was waking up with confusion, requiring periodic pain medications. As expected, he was not moving his right side since a stroke in the left hemisphere of the brain will cause weakness on the right side of the body. His lungs were swollen and full of fluid. Physicians could not take him off the breathing machine. To complicate matters further, his kidneys had stopped functioning such that the nephrologist (kidney doctor) wanted to do dialysis. All this time, his left foot remained in jeopardy.

Patients who develop kidney failure suddenly, like Bill, need emergency dialysis to correct acid, electrolyte, and fluid levels in the body. Diane was worried. What if the kidneys had shut down forever, and what if he needed dialysis all his life? Bill had functioning kidneys before, so recovery was possible. Even so, he had vascular disease, and his kidneys therefore appeared small and scarred on recent images. There was a possibility that he might need dialysis all his life.

Diane remained dutifully at the bedside. Bill's brother had visited and left. Diane was tearful much of the time; she did not understand any of this. Her daughter Liz was angry. Every day they both came in hoping to hear some good news. Would he recover?

How would he recover from multiorgan failure? For any patient who is admitted to the intensive care unit, an outcome or survival score can be calculated. One of these scoring systems is called the Sequential Organ Failure Assessment (SOFA). SOFA considers the function of heart, lungs, and other organs. Each failing organ adds mortality points. Not surprisingly, the worse the multiorgan failure, the higher the likelihood of death. At one point, the mortality rate calculated for Bill was 95 percent, but it had been upgraded with better wakefulness, improved liver tests, and corrected oxygen levels. Now it stood at 70 percent.

Premorbid conditions (the conditions existing *before* the patient is admitted—e.g., lung, kidney, and heart disease) and capacity to function play a huge role in recovery from such devastating multiorgan failure. Some scoring systems take these conditions into account when predicting mortality.

What do the scores mean? What does a 70 percent prediction of death mean?

Mostly, it means that the loved one is very sick. It is appropriate to inform other members of the family that the patient is in critical condition in the hospital and that they should visit if they can. It means that even with expert doctors working to save the patient, death is a real or even likely possibility. A family should come together to support each other and ask for spiritual support or a member of the clergy if they are religious. They can also ask for emotional support from the palliative care team. It is important for families to show inner strength, put away differences, and decide things in the best interests of the patient. It is a time of shock for the family, but most families stay hopeful. Even when doctors prepare the family, repeatedly, the death comes as a blow.

What does a prediction of 70 percent likelihood of death mean? Patients who have had minimal activity or have had many complex diseases before coming into the hospital are likely to fall into the category of patients that die. One example could be a person with significant emphysema who requires oxygen all the time. Another could be a person with extensive heart failure who has barely been getting out of bed. A patient who has had a good level of function before coming into the hospital has a better chance of being in the smaller group of patients who survive. While deciding for aggressive care, this premorbid picture should be kept in mind. Patients' desires regarding long-term care should be borne in mind because all survivors need long-term care, possibly in a nursing home for many weeks.

Diane went through all the normal stages of grief during the days of her bedside vigil: anger, denial, bargaining, depression, and acceptance. With any sudden illness, these emotions are common. However, one phase may last longer than another. Anger, in general, is directed toward the patient, the self, or the medical system. There is often someone or something to blame. Why did he smoke so much? Why did I let him smoke? Why did his coworkers not find him in time? There is a worry that nurses and doctors don't communicate with each other and the family. Nurses heard many of Diane's thoughts over next few days: Bill can never die! He is a fighter. He has come through worse problems. I can't imagine a life without Bill. Unfortunately, the recourses in the health care system to deal with loved ones' enormous depression and stress are insufficient.

Diane was concerned about dialysis but more so about the surgeon's words. The left leg was not viable and was adding to the toxins in the body. They wanted to remove the part of the left leg below the knee. Diane knew Bill would "flip out" if it were amputated. She thought he would hate her for allowing it every day of his life. The doctors said that he would die without the amputation.

Diane, as well as the doctors, knew that Bill could not participate in the decision-making process. Bill was expected to have right-sided weakness and speech difficulties for the long term. He could have additional strokes, particularly if he went to the operating room for leg surgery, but options were limited. Diane wished Bill would wake up and tell her what he wanted. She knew that this proud man was not going to be 100 percent functional. She also knew that he would not want to live being any less; however, the doctors recommended that care continue. She agreed to the surgeries.

The surgeries were successfully completed, and Bill seemed to be healing well. He had lost his left foot and had a tracheostomy tube in his throat and a PEG feeding tube in his stomach. Two weeks later, Bill was moved to a long-term acute care hospital. The tracheotomy allowed the doctors to wean him off the breathing machine. He had a catheter in the neck for dialysis. He was not on any sedative medications and opened his eyes, squeezed with his left hand, and looked around.

Six months later Bill was up and in a wheelchair. He had more strength in his right hand and now some movement in his right leg. His stroke symptoms were improving, though his speech was still affected, and speaking took some time. He no longer needed additional oxygen. The tracheotomy tube, now removed, had left a small scar on his neck. He had a graft in his left arm for dialysis. He went to the dialysis center regularly and took his medications as prescribed. Bill needed pain and anxiety medications. He still liked to smoke, and he said he would make do with the way things turned out.

Eight

Catastrophic event in a patient with chronic disease

Lack of circulation of blood to the tissues of the brain from narrowing of blood vessels causes an *ischemic stroke*. High blood pressure, high cholesterol, smoking, and diabetes are risk factors world over. A *hemorrhagic stroke*, which is caused by a rupture of a small blood vessel, often when blood pressures are very high and uncontrolled, is less common, but with a different presentation and outcome (Figure 8).

Florence had worked at a bar for much of her adult life. She had married several times, but stuck to her cigarettes. She told her family, "I'll quit smoking when I'm dead." Florence had started smoking at a very young age. She had developed emphysema and significant shortness of breath over the years. Now, at the age of 70, she lived at home by herself. Her daughter Candace had focused through all the distractions in their lives and become a nurse.

Florence was indeed limited in her function. She needed oxygen all the time and used her inhalers frequently. She had a tank of oxygen to take along whenever she went outside of the home and had an oxygen concentrator at home. She became short winded with minor activity and could barely finish the chores at home. Despite ill health, Florence was always jovial and funny. Her daughters loved her and checked on her regularly. Sometimes after a huffing spell, Candace would hear Florence say, "One of these days I'll be gone. But you know, I am good with that." All the girls knew that Florence was a relatively independent soul and loved life the way it was. Florence had expressed that she did not want to live connected to machines.

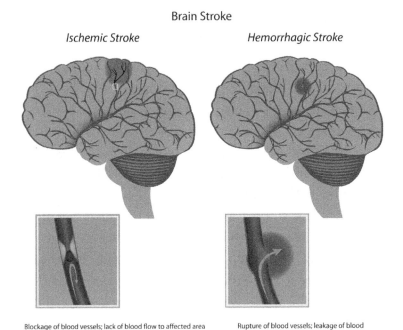

Blockage of blood vessels; lack of blood flow to affected area   Rupture of blood vessels; leakage of blood

Figure 8: Stroke or cerebrovascular accident (CVA)
is a brain tissue blood circulation problem.

Three months before her current hospitalization, Florence experienced fluttering of the heart and felt dizzy. She was examined in a hospital and found to have an irregular rhythm of the receiving chambers (atria) of the heart—a condition called *atrial fibrillation*. Atrial fibrillation allows blood to stagnate and clot within the heart. This clot can dislodge from the heart and travel to various parts of the body, including the brain. It is not an uncommon cause of stroke. Based on the risk factors, blood thinners are recommended for atrial fibrillation. Coumadin is a blood thinner that acts on clotting factors of the blood and is different from aspirin. Newer medications are also available that replace Coumadin. Any blood thinner has its risks and benefits.

One afternoon, the family found Florence on the floor. She was not breathing well, and they called paramedics. The paramedics placed a breathing tube right away. Upon transfer to the hospital, a CT scan of the head was suggestive of a stroke. If a person is found in the first few hours of the attack, the doctors can administer clot-busting medication. The patient may also be treated with a catheter angiogram and clot removal to improve the symptoms of stroke and preserve brain tissue. Time matters.

It is unfortunate that many choose to ignore risk factors for stroke. Avoiding smoking and controlling blood pressure, diabetes, and cholesterol are imperative for long-term health and survival. Many of these things go hand-in-hand with lack of education and poverty. African Americans are more susceptible to having high blood pressure and strokes. The statistics are staggering. This population group has strokes at a much younger age and have higher death and disability rates. Hispanics and Native Americans also have much greater risks. Coronary artery disease and stroke rates are also high among people of Indian subcontinent origin.

Florence's CT scan suggested that a stroke had occurred several hours before presentation; therefore, she was not within the window for receiving clot-buster medication. Florence remained unresponsive and was transferred to the intensive care unit. Her daughters stood next to her; she was now attached to the ventilator. They could see that Florence had no movement on the right side of her body. But the next day, Florence started opening her eyes. She looked to the left side, ignoring the right side. On the third day, she began to move her left side in response to commands, but her right side remained very weak.

While on the breathing machine, Florence's lungs had significant wheezing and secretions. Wheezing sounds are typical for patients with emphysema. Every time the doctors reduced the support of the breathing machine, Florence started breathing fast. Her emphysema was interfering with the reduction of breathing machine support and liberation from it. Ordinarily, doctors wean patients off the breathing machine as they become alert. Once the patients tolerate being weaned to minimal ventilator settings, doctors then check their breathing capacities with an eye toward removing the breathing tube. A physician is always relieved to know that the patient has good alertness, a good cough, and good capacity to breathe without the breathing tube. Given Florence's stroke, as well as her underlying lung problems, there was little feeling of relief.

The daughters sat down with the doctors to decide what to do next. Everybody agreed that Mom had wanted to be independent and free of life support.

Will Florence die from this stroke? The size and the site of the stroke, as well as the swelling of the brain tissue determine if the patient will die in the first few days or weeks or will survive. The National Institutes of Health Stroke Scale (NIHSS) is a tool that hospitals use to assess the severity of stroke. The staff examines a patient with a stroke, documents function and movement, and assigns a particular NIH stroke score. When the presenting scores are very high, the likelihood of death within thirty days is also high. Florence's presenting scores suggested the probability of mortality within thirty days to be as high as 50 percent.

The second part of the question was: *would Florence have reasonable function and be out of the nursing home at the end of three months?* At the time of discharge from the hospital, generally in five to seven days, a modified Rankin score can be assigned to a patient. A patient performing all activities will have a Rankin score of zero or one. Members of the lower Rankin group, with scores of zero or three, have a better scope of recovery. A patient with a Rankin score of five, someone who is bedridden and totally dependent for all their care, is unlikely to recover full function. In other words, if disability after several days of the stroke is devastating, expect poor recovery. Florence had a Rankin score closer to five.

It should be noted that inaccuracy of such scoring systems is routinely criticized. Many scoring systems are inaccurate because they don't take prestroke health conditions into account. Doctors look at the score, then factor in the issues like severe heart failure and thus predict better. Scoring systems predict fine for a 'group' but not as well for an individual.

A specialist who has examined the patient's progress for a few days in the hospital and has seen the scans may be able to make a prediction regarding recovery. Such predictions are in percentages, and how they might apply to an individual patient is tricky to say. Only time can tell how the recovery will unfold. Most patients who do not develop complications will improve slowly, with the greatest improvement during the first three to six months. Beyond this, there can be some—usually limited—recovery.

Candace, along with her other sisters, would have to decide regarding further care. Florence would likely have long-term, right-sided weakness and, given the area of this stroke, would also likely have speech and cough impediments. Even if her lungs sounded completely clean, it would not be clear whether she could protect her airway. Patients with emphysema can get into breathing trouble rather quickly, even with small mucous plugs. To afford her the appropriate time, Florence would need a tracheotomy and very likely need to be on a breathing machine long-term. It was highly probable that at the end of three months, Florence would still be in a nursing home and in a very dependent condition. Could she make remarkable progress? It was possible, but the likelihood was low given the complete picture.

The family knew that Florence would not want a tracheotomy. The other option was to optimize the lung function the best that the doctors could, wait for alertness to improve, and then remove the breathing tube. After that, nature would take its course. If Florence were to improve, she would be offered more therapies; otherwise, she would be provided comfort. The daughters chose the second path. Florence started to open her eyes and look at her daughters. As her wheezing had lessened, she met the criteria for removal of the breathing tube. The family understood that if her breathing got worse, the tube would not be replaced. Florence did okay for a few days after tube removal, with more eye opening and interaction. However, she developed a bout of urinary tract infection, slipping over the next few days. Florence was given comfort medications such as morphine and Valium to see her through her last hours.

Infection and related sepsis (the effect of bacteria or toxins on the body) are among the top causes of admission and death in an intensive care unit. Bacterial overgrowth is common among bed-ridden patients. Once bacteria or toxin enters the blood stream, the body reacts with inflammation and swelling of organs. A septic shock will result in multiorgan failure and death. Severe sepsis strikes more than a million Americans each year. More than a quarter-million may die from this problem— far more than breast cancer, prostate cancers, and acquired immune deficiency syndrome (AIDS) combined.

Candace made the decision with her sisters, considering their mother's wishes and outlook. There was no living will or HCPOA, but the sisters agreed, making the process easier compared with situations where family members disagree with one another. Candace talked to her mom and tried to explain everything. Florence nodded at times; her primary gesture was to pull the tube from her mouth.

Nine

LOW-OXYGEN-RELATED BRAIN INJURY: DRUG OVERDOSE

Letting go

Substance abuse is rampant in all groups in society. Drugs are a cause of death and sickness for young and working-aged populations, but the middle-aged and elderly are not immune. The stories are heartbreaking. Pain medications prescribed by doctors are contributing to the addiction epidemic.

Such is the expectation of the society: complete freedom from pain and pain medication prescriptions on demand. Unfortunately, the body gets habituated to pain medications rapidly, so patients increase the number of pills. Pain control may improve, but by this time side effects are significant and include confusion, sleepiness, constipation, and shallow breathing. Prescribing doctors are unaware of how frequently their patients end up in hospitals due to abuse of their medications. Prescribing narcotics such as Vicodin or Percocet to an elderly patient with back pain may result in a fall and head trauma. Prescribing them to a patient with chronic obstructive pulmonary disease (COPD) may result in respiratory failure. Giving them to patients with kidney or liver disease may result in prolonged confusion. Hospital doctors see this all the time and deal with the consequences.

Terry was only twenty-three but had gone through drug rehabilitation. In high school, he used heroin. Heroin, of course, is highly addictive. Using it a few times at a party can leave teens or adults addicted. Heroin is not often the first drug that kids try. Alcohol, marijuana, and prescription drugs show up at parties much more frequently.

Terry's parents were divorced, and his father lived in Florida. His mother could not cope with his problems, and Terry had had treatment at a rehab clinic in Florida. He was back living with his mother. Terry was partying one night and passed out. His friends thought that he had gone into a deep sleep and did not bother him, but then he started to breathe heavily and started making funny sounds, so they called the paramedics. The paramedics found Terry in a pool of vomit without a pulse, and they performed CPR. Terry received CPR for about twelve minutes before the recovery of a pulse. The paramedics had placed a breathing tube.

Overdose results in suppression of breathing because heroin affects the breathing centers in the brain. Oxygen levels start to drop once breathing becomes very shallow. Oxygen levels must be dramatically low for a significant amount of time for the heart to stop in a young patient. Many states now allow paramedics to carry naloxone (Narcan). This drug reverses the effects of narcotics; however, Terry's case was too advanced for naloxone to work.

Terry was now attached to a breathing machine and in an intensive care unit. He was in a coma. Terry's mom, Rita, was at the bedside. The intensive care unit nurse consoled Rita. When Rita initially received the news, she thought she had lost Terry. Terry had always given her heartache. Every time Rita thought things would be different, it happened again. She had argued, pleaded, and threatened, and then convinced him to go to Florida. Unfortunately, even after rehab, Terry was in the company of the same friends. She was very angry with his friends.

Such scenes are heartbreaking for health care professionals. Lying in front of Rita was her only child—not quite a man, pale, and deadly ill with a tattoo on his neck that read *Mom*. Another tattoo on his arm was a skull with a single word: *death*. Periodically, his whole body jerked, suddenly setting off the alarm on the breathing machine. Nurses came in and gave him medications through the catheters in his veins. Rita held his hand, staring at the multiple puncture wounds on his arms.

The biggest question going through Rita's mind was, "Will he be okay?" Doctors only told her that it was too early to say. They would observe Terry for signs of recovery. His jerking movements were a sign of brain irritability and brain injury. The reduced oxygen levels before and during the cardiac arrest were devastating to his brain. The longer Terry remained in a coma, the worse the outcome. Terry would need to show certain milestones of recovery to indicate substantial progress. In the first three to four days, he would need to start showing an appropriate reaction to pain. Patients who start to open their eyes and look around in the first few days, particularly at the examiner, generally have a good outcome. If the patient remains unresponsive with reduced brain wave response by seven to ten days, they typically do not do very well. Brain scans or electroencephalograms (EEGs) can be helpful, but do not always predict recovery. Continued daily observation is the best way for doctors to predict recovery. The concern of withdrawal from heroin complicated Terry's recovery. He received multiple medications, including opioid narcotics, to keep him comfortable on the breathing machine, but that made examination challenging.

Rita wondered if Terry's heart would stop again. Cardiac arrest was unlikely under the circumstances. The heart is irritable early after an arrest, but a young heart would settle down. Doctors would recommend that the family continue full support for several weeks. CPR may leave the brain further damaged, but was reasonable during the observation period. Doctors would recommend treating infections and low blood pressure during the time of monitoring.

If Terry did not wake up in a week, he would receive a tracheostomy, a feeding tube, and be relocated to a long-term acute care hospital. During this time, observations would be made to see if Terry followed occasional commands or showed signs of organized responsiveness. Even brief purposeful behavior would put him in the category of a minimally conscious state (explained in Chapter 13). If Terry remained unresponsive and nonpurposeful for more than one month, he would be classified as being in a persistent vegetative state. DNR is recommended for vegetative patients at three months. Doctors also ask the family to consider removal of life support if the patient is attached to it. They also recommend not treating infections aggressively. Hospice evaluation is helpful at this stage.

Terry was transferred to the long-term hospital and put on the breathing machine. Over the next few weeks, he had *neurogenic storms*. Profuse sweating broke out, lasting for minutes. His body went rigid, and his heart rate and blood pressure went high. The nurses gave him medications to help this to subside. Rita watched with distress. The breathing machine kept Terry going for some time. Over the next few weeks, doctors successfully got Terry off the breathing machine. Terry had a tracheostomy tube that was attached to simple oxygen tubing.

After Terry had spent many weeks in the long-term hospital with no purposeful activity documented, the long-term hospital could serve no further purpose. Terry was transferred to a nursing home. He stayed off the breathing machine; the tracheostomy maintained his airway. He was treated for a urinary tract infection and pneumonia over the next several months. Rita was upset with the nursing home because she felt they had let him develop a skin breakdown on his buttocks. Terry did not have as many of neurogenic storm events, but he never looked at anybody. His hands seemed to be tightening into fists, and his upper arms were tightening up in front of his chest.

Rita had hoped Terry would someday wake up from the coma. She had heard stories, and she had prayed for a miracle. She had gone through all the phases of grieving. Now she just prayed for peace.

———

Tracy, eighteen years of age, had also suffered brain injury due to cardiac arrest after heroin use. She was still not awake after ten days. The only positive observation for the doctors was that her reaction to pain was now a withdrawal reaction instead of an extension reaction. Withdrawal reaction indicates improved organization of impulse. The next steps of improvement, if they materialized, should be purposeful movement, such as reaching for the tube. Of course, doctors were also looking for opening of the eyes, holding steady eye contact, and following commands.

Tracy's mother, Mary, had been at her bedside holding her hand almost constantly. Nurses noted that Mary had not slept for days. Mary had been through deep mental anguish. She related that drug use had taken an immeasurable toll on her child; she felt in her heart that Tracy was mentally damaged. Even if there were any recovery, she felt that Tracy would never be the same. There was no doubt in her mind that Tracy would almost certainly spend the rest of what time she had at the nursing home, and this thought bothered her: Tracy would never have willingly undergone the indignity of being in a nursing home. If she ever came home by some miracle, would she stay off the drugs? Mary was the only decision-maker; Tracy's father was never in the picture.

Mary had made up her mind: her child had had enough. Mary said, "Doctors, please let her go. My Tracy would never have wanted any of this. She has had enough!"

The doctors did not necessarily disagree with Mary, but they also knew that it was too early to remove the breathing tube. Tracy's state of recovery was not clear; therefore, the doctors

were unwilling to state that Tracy was in a permanent comatose
state. Unfortunately, removal of a breathing tube could possibly
cause demise and equate to withdrawal of care.

A better scenario would be to have Tracy meet parameters
for removal of the breathing tube in accordance with the stan-
dards of medical care. In this manner, the physicians avoided the
withdrawal of care process.

Mary thought that the doctors were not abiding by the wishes of Tracy and Mary. She was upset. She demanded the removal
of the tube. There did not seem to be any possible compromise
between her and the doctors. Everybody agreed that it would be
a good idea to involve the palliative care team and to summon
an ethics committee.

An ethics committee consists of hospital administrators,
medical officers, lawyers, clergy, palliative care nurses, social services, the patient's nurse, and the health care coordinator. The
idea is to listen to the patient (if possible), the family members,
and the health care providers. The goal is to clarify misunder-
standings. Ethics committees give recommendations; these are
not binding.

The ethics committee saw Mary's concerns, but they also
understood the doctors' position and recommended that Tracy
be designated DNR. They asked Mary to give the doctors a few
more days and for Mary to talk to the doctors on a daily basis.
However, if Mary did not like this idea and wanted other opin-
ions or other facilities, the members of the ethics committee
offered to help her find an institution that might offer her what
she wanted. They warned, though, that doctors would likely say
the same thing at most facilities.

Mary agreed to provide more time to the doctors. Tracy's breathing capacity improved a little, and she could tolerate weaning from the breathing machine. Ideally, the patient should be awake and participating in care for the successful removal of a breathing tube, but this is not mandatory if other parameters are met. A few days later, Tracy was removed from the breathing machine. Even so, Tracy was not very responsive. Unfortunately, even after further testing, the neurology and intensive care unit teams could not conclude whether Tracy was going to remain in or slip out of her comatose state. Mary sought hospice assistance. She wanted Tracy home; she did not want any tube feedings. Tracy was discharged home, where she passed away being taken care of by her mother and hospice caregivers.

In this particular case, not surprisingly, there were no advance directives. The patient had been designated DNR at the mother's request. At times, the injury and neurological signs are so poor that physicians have no hesitation in calling a patient terminal. At that stage, doctors and family can sit down to talk about withdrawal of care. Two doctors must sign the paperwork attesting that the patient is terminal. Doctors want all involved family members to be in agreement. Once the doctors and family members sign the document, each institution may have its own requirements regarding wait time and review time before the removal of life support.

Section 3

PROGRESSION TO A TERMINAL CONDITION

Ten

WHEN CANCER TAKES OVER

Taking in the long view

Candi was diagnosed with lung cancer quite unexpectedly; of course, it came as a shock. Candi had been coughing for a few weeks, and she blamed it on the cigarettes. Recently though, cigarettes had been bothering her more than usual, so she had stopped smoking. Initially, physicians thought she had pneumonia; subsequently, a CT scan and then a battery of tests diagnosed her with lung cancer.

The cancer was in the right lung, but it was also affecting part of Candi's breathing tube. There were multiple tumors in her liver. It turned out that she had a stage IV lung cancer. Candi was only 57 and not prepared. She cooked, cleaned, and ran the house as best she could on a modest family income. Her husband was even less prepared and had a meltdown. Her sisters supported her: "We will fight this together. We're going to see you through this, Sis. The good Lord is with us. He will cure you."

But it was not much of a fight. Stage IV lung cancer is an advanced-stage cancer that has spread to other organs, so surgical removal of the tumor was not feasible. Under the circumstances, treatment options were limited. Chemotherapy and radiation may have had initial success, but recurrence of cancer is a problem. Once back at home, Candi's oxygen level was so low and her breathing so shallow that she could barely get around. She was using the oxygen tubing all the time. She could not understand the reason for such a sudden worsening of her condition; this weakness was too debilitating. The doctor had explained that a tumor in her lung was obstructing parts of the breathing tubes so secretions in the airways were keeping oxygen levels low. Pneumonia had left her lungs swollen and her body very weak, but she might recover over time.

Why didn't she start chemotherapy right away? Why wouldn't it cure her? Why wouldn't the doctors start to treat her aggressively? There has been considerable progress in the cure of blood (or *hematological*) cancers. Progress is slow in solid cancers, particularly lung cancer. New treatment plans include novel chemotherapies, immunotherapy, radiation therapies, and surgeries. The key to treatment is diagnosing cancers early. Early stage cancers are easier to treat and the treatments easier to tolerate. It is not surprising that families with better education and resources have better screening than those without. Breast cancer, colon cancer, cervical cancer, skin cancer, and lung cancer screening certainly makes a difference. However, even with the prevalence of screening, more cancers are being diagnosed at advanced stages, when treatment options decrease, reducing positive outcomes and life expectancy.

Doctors were arranging radiation therapy and would arrange chemotherapy when Candi was a little stronger. Even then, the treatment would not offer a cure. It might give her more time. The likelihood that she would still be alive in five years was less than 10 percent. Without treatment, she might have only months to live.

Candi needed to be stronger and free of infection in order to receive chemotherapy and to tolerate it. Chemotherapy is a biological or chemical treatment directed at the cancer cells. However, few chemotherapy agents target only the cancer cells; most affect other functioning cells of the body as well. Chemotherapy can have detrimental effect on bone marrow, the lining of the mouth, hair follicles, nerves, the heart, or any another organ, depending on the type of chemicals. Cancer doctors must make sure that the patient can handle the toxicity. Chemotherapy can reduce the ability to fight infections. There is no sense in administering chemotherapy to a patient who has an active infection. Such a person will die from the infection. That would be premature death, occurring before the cancer would have killed the patient. Additionally, if someone has a weak heart or weak lungs, the toxicity of chemotherapy may not be tolerated.

Cancer doctors check patients' performance status when deciding on, modifying, or predicting the effects of chemotherapy, as well as when prognosticating survival. Performance status is measured on a scale of patient capabilities. The doctors may use one of several scales. In the World Health Organization Performance Status scale, a zero score means unrestricted ability to engage in activity while a score of four indicates a very dependent patient who may not be able to do anything for himself or herself. The likelihood of surviving an advanced-stage cancer may decrease dramatically as the performance decreases. In patients with poor performance scores, cancer doctors may see no benefit in administering chemotherapy unless it may specifically alleviate some pain. Cancer specialists (*oncologists*) would call this *palliative chemotherapy.*

It should be noted that some studies show that patients think the cancer doctors are underestimating their survival. This optimism is a human nature for survival, as well as good and important for recovery. At the same time, it is often a hindrance to acceptance of reality.

Candi had a poor performance status. If it were to improve a little, then she might benefit from chemotherapy. If her level of function remained low, then choosing comfort care or hospice care could have been an option. Candi could not believe that doctors would give up on her. John would not even hear of it. Unfortunately, though, just a week after her release from the hospital, Candi was readmitted. Soon, she was on a mask and receiving the maximum amount of oxygen. It was not that the cancer that had advanced rapidly. Rather, the cancer had caused swollen air passages, collapsing her right lung. That afternoon, the oxygen level was so low that nothing but a ventilator would support her. Candi had expressed wishes to be declared DNR. Her cancer doctor had talked to her about this possibility of rapid decline. He had communicated her options to her. Candi knew she had limited time and did not want life support to be her last memory. Hospice care was her alternative to discomfort.

But her husband, John, would have none of it. He cried, cajoled, and convinced Candi to receive full support. Unfortunately, the breathing machine doesn't alter what's happening to the lungs. Candi now had massive right-lung pneumonia on top of extensive lung cancer. Radiation to her lung was arranged, but her oxygen levels were hard to maintain. Multiple adjustments were made to the breathing machine. Transportation out of intensive care unit to the radiation unit was not feasible. In a few days, John realized that his wishes were causing her misery. She was just unhappy with the breathing tube down her throat. The sisters and family sat down with the palliative care team. Candi communicated to the family that she wanted comfort care.

Why does cancer cause pain? Solid cancer cells are an unregulated mass of cells that keep on multiplying and result in larger growths. The organ in which they are growing, whether it is a lung, a kidney, or the brain, starts to show problems. Small chunks of cells break off and are lodged into nearby lymph nodes or enter the bloodstream and travel to distant organs, thereby causing metastasis (Figure 9). Organs show dysfunction as tumors reach a critical mass. These tumors don't have organized pain receptors, so tumors are not painful, but whichever organ they grow in—for example, a kidney—will have a surrounding capsule, and this is the place with pain or stretch receptors. Constant dull aching or gnawing pain is described. A tumor in the brain causing pressure can cause substantial headache.

Pain is most severe when tumors erode surrounding tissue or invade structures like the bone. The lining that surrounds the bone, the *periosteum*, is painful to stretch; this is an important cause of discomfort. Alternatively, bones can fracture due to tumors and become unstable. Movement of such an unstable bone is very tender. Vertebral and rib cage bones can move and hurt with each breath. Nerve roots can be compressed by the tumor or the fracture, after which slight motion can induce sharp, shooting pain.

Why does cancer cause death? Cancer may contribute to the shutting down of an organ. In Candi's case, it was the lungs. In other cases, the bowel can be studded with tumors, making it impossible to digest food. In the case of the brain, the tumor can cause swelling and increased pressure. Often, the cancer may erode blood vessels, resulting in bleeding in critical structures. At other times, malignant fluid collects around the heart and thus impedes its function.

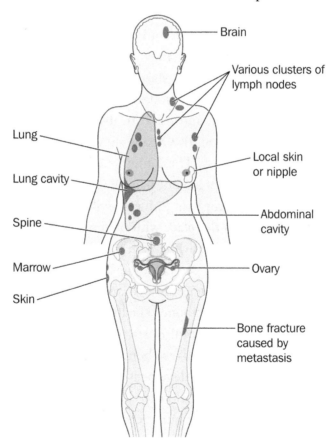

Figure 9: Metastatic cancer. (permission from fotosearch.com)

In certain cases, death is not due to direct involvement of the organ. Instead, the body may become susceptible to infections or blood clots. In addition, chemotherapy may cause side effects, including failure of bone marrow, among other problems. Ultimately, when treatment is not working, cancer overwhelms the body.

If a cancer specialist tells a patient that the options are exhausted and that the patient is terminal, it means the patient often has weeks to a few months to live. In general, cancer doctors are optimists and will provide aggressive therapies as safely as they can. For patients with advanced cancer for whom the additional line(s) of chemotherapy have failed, doctors may offer other palliative treatments. *Palliative* means to reduce discomfort, but the patient and family often construe this to be a line of chemotherapy that will rid the patient of the cancer. In fact, palliative chemotherapy may not bring comfort at all. The chemotherapy may have toxicity (nausea, infection, fevers, etc.), yet the chance of improvement may be slim. The "survival benefit" might be only a few weeks. Some patients might consider these last few days more important and might want them free of toxicity. Focusing on pain symptoms, quality of life, and being free from hospitals is more important to them.

A palliative care team offers an evaluation of the patient's overall status. This expert team talks to patient and families and discusses the prognosis and care preferences. Team members tease out the hopes and goals of care and discuss DNR versus continued care. Additionally, they talk to different doctors to clarify patient questions. Subsequently, they present all the possible options and resources available. Team members see how patients can be made comfortable and assist with hospice care as needed. A palliative care team is a great resource for an ICU doctor because, along with all the other things mentioned above, team members assist with redefining the direction of care. Hospice care can take over comfort care after discharge from the hospital.

Family members may force a patient to keep on going. Often, this is good. Hope is important in this terrible emotional fight that has its ups and downs. Candi did not get much opportunity to fight, but most patients do. Patients should undergo treatments and enroll in trials; and their providers will battle with them aggressively with a goal of best outcome. Some battles will be lost and, when the cancer is becoming overwhelming, every-one should step back and take a long view. Emotions take away the ability to identify the reality of the loved one's circumstances, their pains, and their comfort, and can therefore be the cause of unrealistic expectations.

It is important for patients to have clear communication with their families before a grave illness makes the situation dire. In terminal cases, even when patients and families choose life support, the outcome is often death while the patient is on that life support.

Eleven

BLOOD PRESSURE AFFECTING THE LUNGS: PULMONARY HYPERTENSION

Hope at the end

Emma told her family that she was hopeful. She had just left a top hospital in the country and was so impressed by the doctor. For years, she had suffered from an autoimmune disease called *systemic sclerosis*. She was now on new medications that she hoped would provide good control over her problem instead of losing the battle.

Our immune system is fantastic. It is responsible for identifying foreign cells such as bacteria and for killing them. The immune system does that by producing white blood cells that can kill bacteria in a variety of ways. The immune system can also produce proteins that attach to bacteria and mark them for killing. These immune proteins, known as *immunoglobulins*, can additionally prevent the attachment or replication of bacteria. Immune cells and proteins fight viruses and cancer cells, too.

Asthma and allergies are manifestations of the immune system. In these cases, the system is being hypervigilant. An allergen, like pollen, is greeted with an immune reaction along the lining of eyes, nose, skin, lungs, or bowel. The allergen summons immune cells and proteins in tissues that cause the lining of the eyes or other organs to turn red and weepy.

But, what if immune cells and proteins target healthy tissues of the body as in an autoimmune disease? In this case, the reaction will result in the destruction of healthy tissues. Such is the craziness of the complex systems of the body. Unfortunately, this happens. Many different types of autoimmune disorders have been identified.

Emma had systemic sclerosis. The immune reaction was resulting in deposits of scar tissue along the skin and joints. Her skin was leathery thick in places, and she had difficulty bending her fingers. Her problem became worse when she started to have trouble swallowing her food. The food pipe was becoming thickened with scar tissue and was losing the normal motility that's needed to advance the food down into the stomach.

Not surprisingly, Emma had significant activity limitations. The most dramatic problem, though, was that the disease was affecting her lungs—in particular, the blood vessels of her lungs. The blood pressure in her pulmonary vessels was high. Systemic sclerosis was causing pulmonary hypertension.

When measuring blood pressure, a cuff is placed around an arm. The reading is a measure of the pressure experienced by our organs. This pressure fluctuates as the heart beats, measuring a little higher when the heart chamber (the left ventricle) is actively pushing the blood and slightly lower when the ventricle is at rest. The higher pressure, called *systolic pressure*, is generally around 120 millimeters of mercury (mmHg). The lower pressure, or the *diastolic pressure*, is usually measured around 80 mmHg.

The blood circulating through the lungs (via the pulmonary artery), on the other hand, is pushed by a separate chamber (the right ventricle) at a much lower pressure. The systolic pressure measured in the pulmonary artery is around 25 mmHg, and the diastolic is around 15 mmHg. In the case of Emma, the systolic blood pressure in lungs was nearly 100 mmHg. Therefore, she had severe *pulmonary hypertension*. The strain on her heart due to such high pressures was tremendous, and her shortness of breath was significant. She was using oxygen all the time, and after only a few steps she was exhausted.

Emma had thought of her mortality, and she knew she could not go on forever in this manner. She did not want to live on machines and had communicated this to her daughters, so they created a living will. She had now come to live in Ohio with her daughters, leaving her home in California. Previously, her specialist, a senior rheumatologist (a specialist in autoimmune disease) had taken good care of her, offered all sorts of help, and given her hope. Autoimmune disease is a multiple-organ problem, and doctors from different specialties are required to participate in the care of the patient.

Recently and rather rapidly, Emma's breathing had become very short. Like many diseases described in this book, pulmonary hypertension is a progressive problem. In chronic diseases, the body compensates until a tipping point is reached, and then all compensation mechanisms fail and the patient declines precipitously. The fact is that life expectancy is limited to several years only for patients diagnosed with severe pulmonary hypertension. In later stages, such as in Emma's case, life expectancy is only a few months.

Emma had now seen a specialist in pulmonary hypertension at a very reputable center in Ohio. A new medication had been started. New drugs are available for clinical trials fairly regularly. Centers with such expertise will enroll a qualified patient in a trial and see how its benefits compare to a standard treatment. The effectiveness of the new medication is measured by parameters such as increased number of steps walked or symptoms improved. Some trials measure improvement in survival, generally as weeks or months. Most new medication trials are what they state: trials.

Now back home, even on new medicines, the symptoms were coming back. Emma was feeling so short-winded that she had to go to the emergency room and be hospitalized. By evening, she was breathing harder and needed a BiPAP mask. This BiPAP device, a tight-fitting mask, would provide her with a little pressure pushing air into her lungs. This method sometimes helps prevent the patient from being placed on life support or the ventilator. It was clear to the doctors and her family that Emma was slipping. Earlier, she had declared that she wanted to be designated DNR, but now she felt she needed to see her specialist at the referral center. Emma thought that that doctor would be able to help her. She wanted to be placed on life support, if necessary, to get to that referral hospital. That evening though, that specialist could not be reached by phone, but the covering doctor was willing to provide care if she came to his facility.

After extensive discussions and with the understanding that this might not be feasible or that Emma could die before transfer to the referral facility, the doctors decided to place her on the breathing machine. Unfortunately, once on the breathing machine, Emma's blood pressure dropped precipitously. The possibility of transportation to that facility diminished rapidly. Over next forty-eight hours, despite blood pressure medication support, Emma's heart stopped beating. CPR was not performed. The family was at the bedside. The doctors later spoke with the referral specialist, who said that she had offered no concrete hope to the patient. She had clearly stated that the medication might provide temporary benefit if any. She told the family, as well as the patient, that hospice care would be a good option.

It is not uncommon to encounter a situation where a patient has made a decision to be designated DNR but changes his or her mind. It is also not uncommon for patients under these circumstances to hear what they want to hear. In this particular case, the living will was of no use because the patient remained awake and participated in decision making. Even so, one of the family members questioned if she could have been of sound mind with low oxygen levels. The doctor on call that night had to do his best to understand the situation. If Emma had not been able to participate in decision making, she would have met the criteria for implementation of her living will. She had a terminal condition so the doctors would then focus on comfort instead.

Everyone hopes for a long, healthy, and enjoyable life. It is inappropriate for the medical system to hold out false hope that will cause uncomfortable prolongation of death. Expert doctors put patients on third-tier medications. The patients hear that they are on lifesaving, life-changing drugs and will be cured. In reality, many of these expert doctors are often enrolling patients in trials to see if a medication has any benefit at that stage. *Early involvement of a hospice is crucial for all terminally ill patients.*

In the British system, this burden is placed on physicians. They will tell the spouse or the patient that the case has reached the end of the line, that there is no sense in attempting futile therapy, and that comfort care is a decent option. The downside to that is that a small percentage of patients who may have benefitted from further therapy will not get access to it. In the American system, it ends up becoming a journey of self-discovery. Physicians are supposed to provide intervention and information, even when they know that ultimate choice is unwise. The American focus is on patient autonomy. At the heart of holding out for the next line of therapy is a hope of recovery, however temporary. The expectation is the return to function and possibly to the enjoyment of life, however brief. These positives are countered by the discomfort of dealing with hospitalizations and toxins in the body or the discomfort of disease and medications that might hamper the enjoyment of this brief gain of time.

Twelve

Honoring a patient's expressed wishes

Returning from her mother-in-law's funeral one day, Doris wanted to make sure she did not end up on machines. Her husband Jack, whom she had married thirty years before, was of the same mind. Ten years later, Doris was seventy-six and not as strong. She had been battling rheumatoid arthritis for years and required immune-modifying medications. Rheumatoid arthritis is an autoimmune disorder that causes joint stiffness and deformity. Such destructive scarring can happen in the lungs.

For almost a year, Doris had felt short of breath when active. Her lung physician (*pulmonologist*) performed a CT scan of her chest and a scope examination of her lungs. The CT scan was suggestive of *pulmonary fibrosis*, a progressive scarring disease of the lungs. Her pulmonologist tried steroids for a time, and then gave it up due to the minimal benefit. He offered to refer Doris to a center in a nearby city for expert review, but felt that the immune-modifying drug she took for her rheumatoid arthritis was the best ongoing option.

Pulmonary fibrosis can cause progressive reduction in oxygen levels, thus limiting life expectancy. If lung fibrosis does not respond to any treatment, patients may have only a few years to live. They may die due to low oxygen levels. Doris had been requiring three liters of oxygen per minute almost continuously and complained of swelling in the legs.

Immune-modifying drugs partially suppress the immune system so that the body does not produce antibodies to normal tissues. By the same token, the immune-modifying medications prevent immune cells from acting against infection. Doris had tolerated the medication without problems for quite some time. Now, she presented with increasing shortness of breath. The doctors thought it might have started with a viral pneumonia. Pneumonia flared up in both of her lungs. Apart from pneumonia, the lungs may swell due to a flare-up of pulmonary fibrosis. Doris needed the breathing machine. Her doctors faced a dramatic decline in her oxygen levels, even with the support of the ventilator. The levels were so low the doctors had to use a unique rotating bed. The bed rotated to face downward—so that Doris was facing the floor. After a few hours, the bed rotated around so that Doris faced the ceiling. For two weeks, each day was a battle. Low blood pressures, kidney failure, and fevers required critical, moment-to-moment attention.

Doris survived, and her oxygen levels improved. She completed the course of her antibiotics, and respiratory therapists slowly weaned the breathing machine. However, Doris remained extremely weak and lethargic, barely opening her eyes, occasionally following a command. Her breathing capacity never reached the point where physicians could take her off the breathing machine. It was clear that she would need to remain attached to the breathing machine for a long time, in which case she needed an artificial airway: a tracheostomy. A breathing tube that goes through the mouth is not safe in the long-term, mainly because of potential injuries over time to the mouth and the vocal cords.

Doris's husband, Jack, was a retired engineer. Jack had many valid questions. Would Doris ever get off the breathing machine? Would she be strong enough to go home? Would she be able to eat and enjoy life? He knew she would not want to live long-term in a nursing home. At the same time, he wanted to do everything to keep her going if she would recover. He wanted to understand her chances of survival with long-term support.

Typically, after the placement of a tracheostomy, patients go to a nursing home or a long-term acute care hospital. A long-term hospital is staffed with nurses, speech therapists, respiratory therapists, physical therapists, nutritionists, pharmacists, and doctors just like any regular hospital. Such facilities offer therapy and attempt to wean patients off breathing machines as the circumstances allow. Over time, if feasible, they will try removing the tracheostomy tube. They will focus on rehabilitation and speech therapy in the hope of sending the patient home. The success rates of such hospitals in achieving this goal depend on the conditions of their patients before being admitted. In younger patients, the recovery is faster and success rates higher. If a patient has long-term, disabling lung, heart, or stroke problems, then the success rate may be minimal. For a patient who clearly needs to be moved out of the hospital but is not quite ready to go to a nursing home or home, these facilities provide necessary care. Even though LTAC facilities promise aggressive therapies, not all patients get them. The rate of recovery and home discharge for patients like Doris is usually poor.

Of the patients admitted to an intensive care unit with extensive pneumonia, 20 percent are likely to die. Some patients, like Doris, who develop acute respiratory distress syndrome, can have a probability of death as high as 35 to 40 percent. The likelihood of death in the group of patients who have multiorgan failure can be as high as 80 percent. Of the patients who die, many die in the hospital and others after discharge, in a nursing home or long-term hospital over the next few months.

Doris had survived multiple-organ failure, but her recovery was far from ideal. She still needed a very high percentage of oxygen on the ventilator and had profound lethargy and significantly flaccid extremities. If she went to a long-term hospital after a tracheostomy and feeding tube placement, she would still face significant challenges. Repeat infections in the lungs, skin, urine, and intravenous (IV) lines would be problematic. Such infections might cause irreversible setbacks, death, or result in transfer back to the hospital.

Doris's conversation with her husband was useful regarding tracheostomy, but perhaps even more important in determining the final decision were Doris's ongoing problems before coming to the hospital. The data doctors had on the progression of pulmonary fibrosis was very helpful. Advanced pulmonary fibrosis patients don't do well on ventilator. Without the ventilator, her condition was terminal. With the ventilator, was there a slim chance that she would still be alive in six months? The possibility was small but not zero. Doris would not have a good long-term outlook and would very likely die on the machines, something she never wanted to happen. Two doctors signed the paper for terminal withdrawal of care. So did the family.

It should be noted that doctors are better at predicting poor outcome than at predicting good outcome. Nurses are more pessimistic in outcome prediction than physicians.

Some families and, many times, the doctors are stuck in the "What if she recovers?" scenario. If the family had not agreed with the doctors' recommendations, Doris would have gone to a long-term hospital. In poor survival cases like Doris's, the family faces a long road with no closure. Frustration with poor progress; repeat infections; recurrent hospitalizations; and, ultimately, death hound the family.

Thirteen

Loss of Consciousness: Coma

The notion of a 'fighting chance'

Ariel Sharon's story is more informative than most others. A lot has been written about his life, illness, and death. Israel honored Ariel Sharon highly for his military service. Mr. Sharon became the eleventh prime minister of Israel at the age of seventy-seven. Mr. Sharon enjoyed food, and he was overweight; at 5 feet 7 inches in height, he weighed more than 250 pounds.

It is no surprise that Mr. Sharon lived a busy life and faced day-to-day challenges of the highest order. He had many risk factors for stroke and, not surprisingly, he suffered one. His workup was remarkable in that it revealed an opening between the receiving chambers of his heart—the atria—called a *septal defect*. Doctors put Mr. Sharon on blood thinners for this problem.

On January 5, 2006, he suffered a massive hemorrhagic stroke and was rushed into surgery for evacuation of the blood and reduction of pressure on his brain. Unfortunately, Mr.

Sharon remained in a coma. A coma is a state in which awakening is absent, even with vigorous stimulation of the body. Consciousness of surroundings seems to be missing. Coma does not mean that the body does not react to any stimulation, but rather relates to the inability to be roused and interact. Coma is a sign of brain dysfunction due to injury, drugs, or serious imbalances in a body.

Bleeding and other causes of brain injuries that result in coma can also progress to brain cell death, increased intracranial pressures, and loss of circulation leading to an irreversible cessation of brain function.

If no function of the brain can be detected, brain death is a concern. The medical team must make sure that certain conditions like low temperature, low pH, certain drugs, or other factors are not the cause of this absent brain function.

The core activities of the body—such as breathing, swallowing, and reaction of the pupils—are controlled by the primitive part of the brain called the *brain stem* (Figure 10). Irreversible loss of function of the brain stem is consistent with brain death. Blood circulation to the brain stem is absent in the event of brain death. By the time the flow of blood to the brain stem has stopped, most of the upper brain has already lost its circulation and tissues of the brain have died.

On suspicion of brain death, doctors examine the patient several times and perform different tests to ascertain the function of the brain stem. They will look for even the minutest ability of the patient to breathe and even check for the circulation of blood through the brain stem. If doctors are confident that the patient is brain dead, they will pronounce the patient as having passed away. This is a situation of death while the heart is still beating. It is often hard for families to understand. At this stage, doctors will remove all life support, as dictated by state laws. The family might choose to donate organs at this juncture if that was patient's wish. Since a beating heart preserves the tissues, organ donation is much more feasible.

HUMAN BRAIN

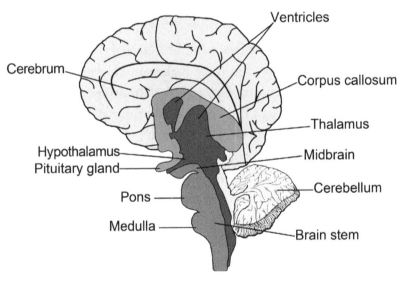

Figure 10: The higher brain, the cerebrum, processes information; parts of the brain stem maintain body functions such as breathing. (permission from fotosearch.com)

The doctors were worried that Mr. Sharon's condition might progress to brain death. Having said that, in both Judaism and in Islam, there are philosophical and religious concerns regarding the pronouncement of brain death, as well as subsequent organ donation. Mr. Sharon did not meet the criteria for brain death, as he had brain stem function. No doubt, his cerebrum had suffered grievous injury. The cerebrum (the "new brain" or "neo-brain") is the site of higher brain function. Thoughts, orientation, and understanding of the environment happen here. Interpretation of consciousness happens here. It defines a person.

Mr. Sharon's two sons were the decision makers. They wanted him to have a fighting chance of recovery; he had been a fighter all his life, after all. Mr. Sharon underwent a tracheotomy and feeding tube placement and was carefully supported on machines for years. He had some eye opening, but beyond this, whether he ever responded to commands is debated. Many tests, including MRIs, were performed to ascertain Mr. Sharon's brain function. His sons believed that he had some underlying consciousness. The family remained hopeful that one day he would become interactive. A particular type of MRI scan called a functional MRI looks at the areas of the brain that light up in reaction to certain kinds of stimulation. A functional MRI may tell if a patient is properly processing information in certain parts of the brain. If Mr. Sharon had occasional appropriate responses— that is, recognizing sounds and trying to move or speak in reaction—he might have been in a "minimally responsive state." In such a case, there may have been hope of recovery.

After waiting for more than a year, the Israeli government declared Mr. Sharon permanently incapacitated. His successor, Ehud Olmert, was then promoted to prime minister. Some believed, though, that Mr. Sharon was in a *vegetative state*.

A vegetative state is an irreversible state of absence of awareness and response. The deep primitive part of the brain remains viable, and many motor reactions are present. The patient may look around, have sleep cycles, and yawn. However, the neo-brain is severely and permanently damaged. As mentioned, the neo-brain makes us who we are, gives us personality, helps connect our memory, and makes us understand stimuli. A patient in a vegetative state lacks any self-awareness or awareness of his or her surroundings. There is no recovery of function. *Anoxic* or *hypoxic* brain injury (injury related to low oxygen, as with heart arrest, stroke, etc.) and trauma are leading causes of a vegetative state.

If a patient remains in a coma for one month after a stroke or low-oxygen injury (as in Mr. Sharon's case), doctors call it a *persistent* vegetative state. At three months, they call it a *permanent* vegetative state.

Trauma is different. Doctors like to observe for a year before they conclude that the patient will remain in a permanent vegetative state. Trauma recovery is different from anoxic recovery because the mechanism of cell injury and death is different. In particular, the recovery from axon injury in trauma is difficult to predict. The primary purpose of watching the patient before designating them as being in a permanent vegetative state is to make sure that they are not in a minimally responsive state.

Most people in America say they wouldn't want to live in a vegetative state. The burden of observation of patients under these circumstances is huge. Many remain on a ventilator for months. As mentioned before, urine, lung, and skin infections, as well as skin breakdown and contractures are typical. However, the family may not "let go," even when the evidence is clear that there is no scope of recovery. There may be guilt in some cases because of the accident, or they may have deep religious convictions, or perhaps simply can't let go. If one asks family members if they would you want to live like this, they invariably say, "No."

It should be noted that there is apprehension among some that the medical system may have cost-saving benefits in mind in not wanting to offer this observational care. The worry is that families are given a poor prognosis and encouraged to limit care. There is suspicion that hospital systems that depend upon insurance reimbursements and that physicians who depend upon bonuses, may have conflicts of interest in providing prolonged care.

At the age of eighty-five after being in a coma for years, Mr. Sharon had undergone abdominal surgeries. He developed kidney problems that worsened in January 2014. Mr. Sharon needed dialysis for the loss of his kidney function. Some debate must have taken place among family and physicians. Would there be a real benefit with dialysis?

Mr. Sharon did not have any advance directives. His family made judgments on his behalf. Maybe that is what he had conveyed to his sons. He passed away on January 11, 2014, after spending eight years in a coma.

Section 4

Organ Failure Causing
Limited Life Expectancy

Fourteen

Smoking-Related Lung Disease: COPD

Determined to keep on going

Smoking-related lung injury is a whole spectrum of diseases. One of the diseases associated with smoking is called chronic obstructive pulmonary disease (COPD). COPD can manifest as emphysema or chronic bronchitis. Patients and families hear these terms from doctors. Emphysema is a process of slow damage, loss of elasticity, and loss of lung tissue leading to shortness of breath and low oxygen levels. Chronic bronchitis is a persistent swelling of the lining of the windpipe and its branches, the bronchial tree (Figure 11). Frequent infections called *bronchitis* are common. Shortness of breath, low oxygen levels, and strain on the heart are usual.

COPD is the third-leading cause of death and disability in the United States. Unfortunately, young people get hooked on smoking early in their lives, believing they are invincible and immune to COPD or lung cancer. Out of one hundred people who start smoking, twenty will develop COPD. Considering the older smokers who have *continued* to smoke, almost 50 percent of smokers will eventually show signs of COPD. Many develop COPD because of environmental factors. The vast majority of patients with COPD are undiagnosed or underdiagnosed, making the problem even worse.

Chronic Obstructive Pulmonary Disease (COPD)

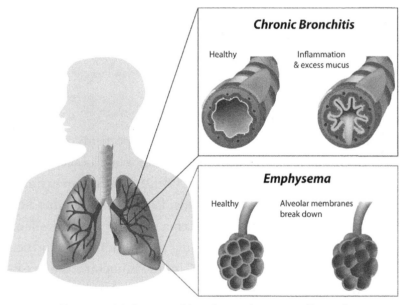

Figure 11: Medium-sized breathing tubes get swollen and infected in chronic bronchitis, while emphysema is a disease of the air sacs. (permission from fotosearch.com)

Edward was diagnosed with COPD many years ago. He wheezed heavily going from his bed to the kitchen. Periodically, he just sat down and grabbed an inhaler for puffs of medication.

He woke up in the morning coughing and spitting up gobs of phlegm. Once or twice a year, Edward developed an atrocious spell of lung tightness that was not relieved by breathing treatments and resulted in hospitalization. He had gone through many courses of antibiotics and many courses of the steroid prednisone. Prednisone increased his sugar levels and made him feel restless.

Edward was seventy-seven years old and had lived with COPD long enough to know how to manage, but it was still a challenge. He had quit smoking two years before, on his seventy-fifth birthday. His pulmonologist told Edward that his breathing capacities were about 30 percent of what would be expected of a healthy male his age. Edward had stage IV COPD. In stage IV COPD, the body weight decreases and malnutrition sets in as the body loses proteins and muscle mass; the skin loses elasticity, appearing thin. Edward's oxygen levels were low, so he required a portable oxygen tank, which he carried around, and at night he kept an oxygen concentrator at his bedside. This oxygen was the crutch he needed to carry on. With it, he could do more and felt a little stronger.

"How long do I have, Doc?" Edward would ask. Even when patients have significant emphysema, the probability of surviving for one year is high. Home oxygen often helps. Cessation of smoking is the most relevant life-improvement move that COPD patients can make for themselves. Patients who have quit smoking for many years start to show some improvement in lung function and lung health. They get fewer infections and suffer fewer episodes of wheezing. Smoke is so damaging to the arteries that it is considered an even worse risk factor than cholesterol for heart problems. Heart disease is very prevalent in smokers. So, what causes death? It might be an infection like a pneumonia, or it could be a heart attack. Lung cancer and respiratory failure are other causes of death in someone with severe COPD.

Let's try to answer Edward's question from an observer's perspective. The average life expectancy for an adult male in the United States is seventy-eight years. A life-limiting condition like COPD reduces life expectancy by eight to ten years. Edward probably did not have a very long life ahead of him at his age of seventy-seven years. If Edward were to check with a local hospice agency, the agency would inform him that significantly limited function, oxygen need, frequent admission to the hospital, and heart failure all lead to a relatively reduced life expectancy and are indications for hospice care.

It should be noted that some have concern regarding implementation of a DNR order. For example, a patient may not want CPR for cardiac arrest given poor health, but may be fine with temporary intubation for respiratory failure. Appropriate documentation in the DNR form avoids any questions. An additional worry is that a patient who is designated DNR is given less aggressive care and has a higher chance of death on hospitalization due to the perceptions of the providers.

Edward was in poor shape, but he was managing his life. He had told his doctors and his family to place him on a breathing machine if needed. In fact, Edward had been put on a breathing machine twice in previous years. Both times, he had come off the breathing machine and slowly inched his way back to his previous level of function. If he could come back again like that, Edward felt CPR was acceptable, too.

That brings us to the current story. Edward came in with respiratory failure and a severe bout of pneumonia. Again, he was intubated. Nurses saw him struggling slightly on the breathing machine and gave him medications for pain and comfort. (The ICU was not Edward's favorite place, particularly with the tube down his throat, as he later told his pulmonologist.) Alarms on the breathing machine went off frequently as he coughed and, unfortunately, the breathing tube made him do just that—cough. But, that was not the only alarm; Edward felt like there must have been a hundred different alarms in the devices around him. The pressure cuff on his arm went off as soon as he tried to close his eyes. If it wasn't that, then it was the pressure stockings on his legs that inflated. And, if he could ignore both of those, then it was one of the health care professionals wanting to talk to him, check his vitals, or draw blood. He had lost count of his visitors; there were nurses, care technicians, doctors, respiratory therapists, physical therapists, and phlebotomists. How many doctors did he have? His hands were tied much of the time because caregivers did not want Edward to pull out his tubes by mistake. He had no desire to take a bath, but he got one every day. A temporary feeding tube going down his nose into his stomach was a cause of constant consternation but a necessary evil, delivering nutrition and medication into his gut. And though he never wished diarrhea on his worst enemies, Edward felt it might be better than the condition of severe constipation.

Patients suffer from constant stress and startle reactions in an intensive care unit. They need heavy medication for comfort. It is no surprise that intensive care unit patients suffer from long-term anxiety similar to post-traumatic stress, even after discharge.

Edward was alert, however, and most of the time jotted down notes for his visiting daughter. On the fourth day, the pneumonia changes on his chest x-ray were slightly better. He was not wheezing that much. Unfortunately, his oxygen levels remained dismal. He had dissatisfactory breathing capacity tests for possible removal of the tube and thus couldn't be weaned off the ventilator. Edward was back on full support from the breathing machine.

On the 13th day, all concerned agreed that Edward needed a tracheostomy for further care, and he understood what was needed. Edward's family signed the consent form, and surgery was scheduled for next day. He tolerated this surgery well. At the same time, a feeding tube—the PEG—was placed in his stomach. Subsequently, Edward was transferred to a long-term hospital. He stayed there for almost five weeks. At the end of that time, he was breathing on his own. The therapists at the long-term hospital could liberate him from the breathing machine, but the tracheotomy tube was kept in place.

As the next step, doctors started to put a special valve on the tracheostomy tube, allowing him to speak and swallow food. Ultimately, the tracheostomy tube was plugged. Now, all the air was moving through Edward's mouth and nose. He was breathing and talking through his own airways, and the tracheostomy was no longer needed. The tracheostomy tube was removed and so was the feeding tube, since Edward was now eating well on his own. The therapies were working well. He was ultimately discharged home on five liters (L) of oxygen per minute.

A swollen prostate had hampered Edward's recovery process. A Foley catheter used to drain urine during his hospital stay had left him unable to pass urine. Doctors had removed and replaced the Foley catheter several times. Ultimately, he had a slow recovery with periodic catheter placement. This was an unpleasant experience Edward would have gladly avoided.

Back home, Edward experienced slow progress. He emitted a little whistling sound every time he exerted himself to breathe in. The tracheotomy had left part of his trachea weak. Instead of his windpipe being rigid, now a portion of the pipe was flopping in when he made an extra effort to breathe. Sometimes that was uncomfortable. On his next visit to the doctor's office, Edward seemed to be in good spirits. When asked if he would do it all over again, he said, "Only if the breathing machine was for a few days." If it came to a tracheostomy again, he would not do it. Edward knew that the subsequent infection was going to be harder to shake. He realized that his weak trachea was making his cough ineffective. Every morning he was working twice as hard to get rid of the phlegm.

Edward was now looking at a possibility of an assisted living facility. He was not quite ready for a community DNR, perhaps later, when he could not get out of bed.

Edward probably considered a question we all must face, "Can I *ever* be ready for the inevitable?" or conversely, "Can I *always* be ready for the inevitable?"

Fifteen

Misinterpretation of wishes

Robin Williams's acting career was amazing. He died at the age of sixty-three. Reportedly, he was so depressed that he took his own life. Initially, he was thought to have a Parkinson's-type disease. Parkinson's disease affects the nervous system, causing stiffness of muscles, tremors, and problems with balance. Depression and anxiety are both common in Parkinson's disease. Medications can control many of the symptoms, and thus patients may enjoy reasonable function and capacity. Surgical options may provide relief in some severe cases. In advanced cases, patients may have difficulty swallowing food. The actor Michael J. Fox has been a spokesperson on behalf of research for Parkinson's disease.

Robin Williams's problems were entirely different. Indeed, an autopsy of the brain revealed Lewy body dementia, a less common cause of dementia. Lewy body dementia is hard to recognize because of a myriad of strange symptoms. Lewy body dementia can cause a shuffling walk and tremors, as in Parkinson's disease. Additionally, it causes some symptoms seen in Robin Williams: he was noted to be distracted, unfocused, and profane in many interviews. His wife had described confusion and visual hallucination. With dementia, there is a loss of concentration and, ultimately, the ability of mentation (thinking, solving problems, insight, personality, functioning, and living day-to-day life). A protein called the Lewy protein is deposited in the brain cells, impeding their function. Some of these symptoms may be missed in someone fighting drug addiction. Mr. Williams had problems with addiction to drugs and alcohol, but he was sober at the time of his suicide.

Alzheimer's disease is the most common cause of dementia among older adults. *Beta-amyloid* and *neurofibrillary tangles*, types of abnormal protein deposits, prevent normal brain function. Early symptoms are memory loss, inability to learn new information, and difficulty with orientation. Wandering away and the inability to handle money may progress to hallucination and delusions (a firm belief in something that may be false). Ultimately, a late stage of the disease will result in nonrecognition of self or others and, perhaps, in cessation of eating. The Alzheimer's Association is an excellent resource for families. The Association notes that of 5.3 million people who have Alzheimer's disease, nearly 66 percent are women. The number of patients will increase as the baby boomers age. By 2050, another American may develop Alzheimer's every thirty-three seconds, according to the Alzheimer's Association. The burden on families who care for Alzheimer's patients is tremendous.

Mike was brought to the hospital for a third time in one year. He was ninety-nine years old and had a diagnosis of *organic dementia,* or *vascular dementia.* He had probably had multiple minor or major strokes, affecting the mentation functions of his brain. Mike had been in a nursing home for several years and was periodically visited by a niece. One afternoon, he was less responsive than usual and was brought to the hospital emergency room. He was admitted to the intensive care unit because his sodium level was extremely high. Looking back through his charts, he had been admitted many times due to dehydration and urinary tract infections. He had a feeding tube placed several years ago because he did not eat well. According to reports, Mike was able to say his name and take a few bites of food offered by the staff. He had a small ulcer on his leg, possibly caused by pressure from being in the bed. Otherwise, his skin was free of pressure ulcer. His extremities were stiff from not moving for a long time. There was a phone number of a niece listed in the chart, but the doctor could not get in touch with her.

Mike was a full code at the nursing facility. Unfortunately, Mike became progressively less responsive over the next twenty-four hours. Mike could not maintain his ability to cough, due to lethargy. His oxygen levels prompted significant concern. When the oxygen level could no longer be maintained, doctors had no choice but to place Mike on the breathing machine. They tried to contact the niece, the only listed relative on the chart, but were unsuccessful. Mike was now on the ventilator. Ultimately, the niece was available to talk to doctors on the phone. She confirmed that everything should be done to save her uncle's life, including life support as needed.

The doctors continued aggressive care; slowly, Mike's electrolyte levels improved. Initial symptoms of pneumonia improved, as did kidney function. But, when it came to reducing and removing the breathing machine, Mike did not have the ability to cough to bring up secretions. It was clear that Mike needed long-term ventilator support.

In the meantime, Mike started to face new problems. His feeding tube, which had been placed several years ago, had some leakage around the hole in the stomach wall. Over time, the hole had become larger and some of the stomach juices were leaking around the tube. Changing the size of the tube did not fix the problem. At issue was the motility of the bowel, a common problem in an intensive care unit. Normal function of stomach and bowel was hampered, resulting in a distended abdomen. Mike seemed uncomfortable; his niece, worked at a local university, believed that holding his hand and pulling it upward always relieved his discomfort. She insisted that her uncle was going to live to an age of one hundred years.

After a few days, Mike started to open his eyes, his lungs cleared up, and secretions were reduced. Mike's capacity improved enough to get off the breathing machine. The success was short-lived, however; in two days, the secretions in the lungs increased, and he started to struggle again. Therapists were now suctioning through his nose almost every hour to keep the lungs clear. The experience is not pleasant for any observer, let alone for the patient. His wrinkled face with bushy white eyebrows contorted in pain. The secretions were large, and Mike would not cough. He was not going to keep on going like this. The chest x-ray was getting worse. Very soon, the only option was going to be to put the patient back on the breathing machine. Doctors sat down with the niece again. What were the goals of care?

From the doctors' perspective, Mike had been at a nursing home with a fair degree of dementia and in a bedridden state. Mike ate poorly in bites, at the age of ninety-nine. Now, he was declining with pneumonia and multiorgan effects, often the natural way we die. The niece said that she had heard from Mike that he was going to live to be one hundred. She told the doctors that he had wanted everything done to keep him alive. She said he had been a fighter, and he would fight this, too.

Health-care professionals want to be nonjudgmental but also want to know they are doing the right thing for the patient. The patient is their primary responsibility, not the next of kin. The doctors were clear that patients with advanced age and dementia don't do well.

Mike was not an appropriate candidate for the intensive care unit. Intensive care units are not designed for prolongation of death or discomfort. Physicians wanted to make sure that the niece had thought through the idea of continued aggressive care for Mike. When insisting on such care, families should keep in mind that providers want to enjoy their profession of healing. The community entrusts providers with costly resources. It is their responsibility to use resources on right patients at the right time.

The niece did have appropriate health care power of attorney, and the hospital attorneys reviewed it. The document must have been drawn up by the patient, apparently when he was of sound mind and capable of doing so. Strangely, there was no living will. The doctors ultimately placed Mike back on the ventilator. He did poorly for first forty-eight hours, and his blood pressure then bounced back. He did better on a new set of antibiotics. Soon, the lungs sounded better, and Mike was opening his eyes again. His chest x-ray and breathing capacities were good enough to take him off the breathing machine again, which was removed.

Mike was observed in the intensive care unit for the next few days. On the day he was supposed to move out of the intensive care unit, he started to run a fever. This resulted in new IV lines, more blood sent for cultures, a chest x-ray, change of urine catheter, and repeat culture of urine. Again, Mike started to decline. The nurse administered blood-pressure-supporting medications—vasopressors—off and on. On attempting to reduce these drugs, Mike's blood pressure would be low. After many days of being in the intensive care unit, Mike was getting nowhere. After two weeks, the lungs took another dive. He would need the machine again.

At this point, the conversation with the niece focused on long-term support with a tracheostomy. An artificial airway would result in long-term clearance of secretions. The niece did not agree to the procedure. Even if she had agreed, most surgeons would have an ethical concern with such a surgery. Nor did she agree with transfer to a long-term hospital. By the same token, the long-term hospital representative had evaluated the patient and did not accept the patient because the agency was worried about providing appropriate care, given the niece's stances.

An ethics committee meeting was summoned. The ethics committee sat down with the niece and other health care providers. In the meeting, the niece expressed the belief that Mike would improve. The niece did not want a tracheotomy done, and she did not agree to a long-term hospital transfer. There was no clear solution. The committee told the doctors that they might delegate care to other physicians or transfer care to another facility if they did not feel they could provide ethical treatment. The committee told the niece that she could look for other doctors or find another facility if she thought that Mike would get better care.

Mike was supported until his symptoms started to improve. Mike improved enough to be transferred to the step-down unit. He had ups and downs during this period. Several courses of antibiotics were given. Mike and his providers dealt with urine infections. Nose bleeding was an intermittent problem due to a need for suction through the nose. Transfer back to the nursing home was not feasible due to the continued need for high oxygen levels and an advanced level of care. Mike stayed in the hospital for months, and he made it to one hundred years. One day, he had a cardiac arrest and could not be resuscitated.

This case is uncommon but shows multiple problems with designating health care power of attorney. Maybe the HCPOA designee did what Mike desired. The recommendation is to have a living will, along with HCPOA. A living will trumps HCPOA designation. If doctors had determined that Mike was terminal, they would have honored the living will and provided comfort, and the HCPOA could have been overridden.

Would this happen in other countries?

Mona had advanced dementia, but her daughters had provided all their love and support. Mary was the elder; she had changed jobs. Now, she lived with Mona and worked from home. Caring for Mona had become harder over the last year. Mona had stopped recognizing her daughters. She sat in one place for hours, did not accept food sometimes, and often resisted bathing and changing. Neither sister wanted a nursing home for their mother (there are only a few "dementia unit" nursing homes) and were determined to do everything in their power to care for Mona at home. It was exhausting. Mona had stepped out one day and was nowhere to be found for hours. Mary was in a panic and had to call the police. Her sister, Susan, came over on weekends to help.

Both sisters were clear that Mona would not undergo any heroics or aggressive care. Mona's physician had felt the community DNR was appropriate. Paperwork was pending. A bracelet instructing that the patient was DNR was soon to be worn by Mona. A paper declaration of her DNR status would be put on the refrigerator.

Susan was watching her mom that afternoon when Mona fell. Susan panicked, and she called 911. Mona had been bleeding around the eye, and her breathing was shallow. The paramedics came and started to transfer her to the local emergency room. On the way, Mona's breathing became shallower, so the paramedics put her on a ventilator.

The daughters were outraged and frustrated when they realized that Mona was on life support. They wanted to know why this was done even with the community DNR in place. The emergency room doctors realized that this should not have happened. They removed the tubes at this stage. Mona improved over the next few days and was discharged home.

In this particular case, even though advance directives were in place in the form of a community DNR, the status had not been completely instituted. A bracelet on Mona's wrist would have been helpful. The family members must clearly state to the paramedics that the patient is DNR. If paramedics come in an emergency situation, they do whatever needs to be done to save the patient. They would normally do CPR or place a breathing tube if needed. The only time they would not do this is if the patient is obviously dead, has rigor mortis, or has suffered decapitation. The community DNR is a valuable, yet underutilized tool.

Sixteen

HEART FAILURE

The next big fix

A failed heart is one that can't meet the demands placed upon it. Heart muscles can be weakened by a heart attack (myocardial infarction, or MI) or by a host of other problems, including viruses that can directly damage muscles. On other occasions, it is a bad heart valve causing extra strain on the muscles. When the pump becomes weak, blood flow to organs decreases, kidneys function poorly, and watery fluid collects in the legs and lungs. Shortness of breath, weakness, and congestion of the liver become problematic.

At age sixty-two, Ken had suffered previous MIs. He also had congestive heart failure, Ken's wife said that his heart function was at 30 percent. This is how families phrase it, but this is actually the 'fraction' of blood ejected with each heartbeat. If 100 cubic centimeters (cc) of blood were in Ken's left ventricle at the beginning of a heartbeat, he would pump out 30 cc of that blood into circulation with each beat. (A normal heart may pump out 70 cc per beat).

A stent had been placed in the past, and more recently, Ken was started on a heart-regulating medication (Amiodarone) for atrial-fibrillation. He became short of breath while climbing stairs and suffered swelling of the legs. Being overweight did not help. Ken's cardiologist had placed a dual-chamber pacemaker in the hope of helping Ken's heart.

Ken had been sleeping on the couch recently because lying in bed made him cough. He had been diagnosed with sleep apnea, but he did not want to wear a continuous positive airway pressure (CPAP) mask while sleeping. Ken was found collapsed in the kitchen. When his wife found him, he was not breathing, and she tried CPR. Paramedics arrived and found Ken in cardiac arrest. He underwent CPR for about ten minutes prior to recovery of a pulse. Ken was rushed to the emergency room, where his blood pressure was unstable. He was placed on life support.

Ken did not wake up in the emergency room. Coma after arrest is common. Cooling of the body down to 93 °F is standard practice after cardiac arrest (though it may change). This is in the hope of keeping the tissues of the brain cooler, thus minimizing the damage caused by a low-oxygen state. Over the next twenty-four hours, cooling was stopped. Indeed, the tests suggested a heart attack. The heart rhythm was unstable, and Ken needed blood-pressure medication support. These vasopressors boosted his pressure up. An echocardiogram (echo), a type of ultrasound of the heart, suggested an ejection fraction of 10 percent. Cardiac shock with a heart attack has a grave outlook. The majority of patients in this situation die. Heart catheterization is offered to patients with improving alertness. A stent to open the artery may make the difference. Heart-assist devices may keep the blood flowing.

Ken's kidneys were failing. Unfortunately, he remained in a coma even after five days of observation. Doctors painted a grim picture around the likelihood of recovery. Ken had never discussed these issues with his family. His wife thought that he would probably not want ongoing support. The palliative care team sat down with the family. They discussed the patient's and the family's wishes.

Even initially, when Ken was diagnosed with heart failure and an ejection fraction of 30 percent, his life expectancy was limited. One year after the onset of symptoms of heart failure, 78 percent of patients are still alive; at five years after, less than 50 percent of patients are alive. Patients with uncontrolled symptoms die earlier. The New York Heart Association (NYHA) Functional Classification rates the severity of symptoms. An NYHA Functional Classification level of four means the patient feels shortness of breath even while resting. Members of this group of patients have the possibility of dying within six months. Kidney disease, uncontrolled diabetes, and lung problems reduce life expectancy even further.

So, what causes death? Ineffective heart muscles will result in failed organs, such as the kidneys and lungs. As the disease gets worse, patients are frequently admitted to the hospital with fluid building up in the lungs and with respiratory failure, requiring a BiPAP device or ventilator. Weak heart muscles are susceptible to irregular heartbeat, ventricular fibrillation, and cardiac arrest.

Heart doctors administer a variety of medications to support the heart muscles, keep fluid buildup at bay, and prevent irregular rhythm. They will place pacemakers and defibrillators to prevent dangerous heart rhythms and improve life expectancy and function.

Few doctors talk about the reality of this problem. The cardiologist had not talked to Ken about the limited outlook and did not encourage a review of his wishes. Doctors engage in one therapy after another to prolong life without letting patients understand that heart failure is a life-limiting disease. If close to 50 percent of patients die within five years, the sheer number of patients (six million) with heart failure makes for a large group of patients with an expectation-reality mismatch in terms of outcome. If the treatments are not controlling symptoms, the quality of life and goals of care should be reviewed. Is shortness of breath constant? Are the organs failing? With multiple hospitalizations, the recommendation is to involve palliative and hospice care. Palliation improves quality of life. The possibility of community DNR should also be considered.

O n the other hand, Nick, who was seventy-eight years old, was very functional. He walked a mile every day—on the treadmill in winter. His wife said he was an avid reader and enjoyed his grandkids. They both had living wills and knew that long-term life support was not what they wished. Nick had had a previous small heart attack. He took aspirin every day.

Nick had not counted on having a big heart attack one morning and landing in the intensive care unit. His heart was pumping so weakly that fluid was building up in his lungs. The situation was so bad that he needed the support of a breathing machine. Soon thereafter, he suffered a cardiac arrest with ventricular fibrillation and required a shock and brief CPR. He was placed on medications to control his heart rhythm. Unfortunately, he got very confused and delirious. He was pulling on the tube, so he was given sedative medications and tied down.

Mary, his wife, was very upset and said that he would not want any of this. She wanted life support removed and for him to be "let go." Heart doctors had offered heart catheterization, but Mary refused. Over the next few days, the fluid from the lungs cleared up, and the heart rhythm was stable. Along with that, Nick's alertness improved, and he was weaned down to minimal setting on the ventilator. His breathing capacity was perfect, and the respiratory therapist took him off the breathing tube. The next day, while sitting up in a chair eating his breakfast alongside the bed, Nick talked to the heart doctors. He agreed to heart catheterization and to stents if needed.

Nick was home soon. He continued to have good capacity and he still enjoyed walks. At the next visit, he had a repeat heart echo. The cardiologist had previously hinted that Nick might need an implantable defibrillator. An automated implantable cardioverter defibrillator (AICD) is a device placed in the chest that delivers a shock if the heart goes into ventricular fibrillation. However, Nick did not need it.

Nick's is a case where the patient had a living will and had expressed his wishes clearly to his family. In this case, his wife thought it was time to implement the living will. For the doctors, though, Nick did not quite meet the implementation criteria of the living will. Immediately after an arrest, things may look grim, but frequently heart function settles down. It is important to allow doctors to assess the prognosis and provide standard medical care appropriate to the situation.

Seventeen

Consideration of the quality of life

Helen, aged fifty-five, had been admitted to the hospital two days before with bleeding. Now, her daughters wanted to know more about her condition. They lived in a nearby town, whereas their mother lived with a friend. Helen had been drinking for years and had developed a yellow tinge to her skin. She was also building up fluid in her abdomen. Helen knew that she had cirrhosis: a doctor had told her so a few years before, so she had never gone back.

Alcohol is toxic to the liver cells. A sudden, massive injury to the liver because of an alcohol binge is called *alcohol hepatitis*. Jaundice, nausea, and fevers may develop along with abnormal liver test results. Heavy alcohol use may result in repeated injury to the cells of the liver. Over time, liver cells may die and be replaced by regenerated cells and by scars. The structure and function of the liver change over time; this leads to cirrhosis.

Heavy use is often defined as thirty-two to forty-eight ounces of beer, which is three to four cans of 5 percent alcohol beer, daily, or it could be sixteen to thirty-two ounces of 12 percent wine. Three to four shots, which amount to 1.5 ounces of 40 percent alcohol, would also qualify as heavy daily alcohol use. Significant alcohol consumption over ten to fifteen years can lead to cirrhosis of the liver.

One day, Helen was not feeling well. She had been drinking the previous night. In the morning, she threw up, and there was a significant amount of blood in her vomit. When it happened the second time within the next 15 minutes, she panicked and called the paramedics. At the emergency room, she received blood transfusions. Her blood pressure was low and so was her hemoglobin level. She was admitted to the intensive care unit, and the stomach doctors (gastroenterologists) passed a scope down her food pipe (esophagus) to evaluate the bleeding. Doctors found swollen vessels (*esophageal varices*) all along Helen's food pipe and applied bands in the hope of stopping the bleeding (Figure 12).

Blood flows through the liver unhindered, but when the liver is scarred this can't happen. Backed-up blood induces pressure on veins in the stomach and esophagus. Veins under increased pressure (varices) in the esophagus rupture easily and may cause massive bleeding.

The liver is responsible for the breakdown and synthesis of many substances in the body. Clotting factors and platelets are depleted in cirrhosis, so the bleeding is significant and unchecked. The quantities of many substances, such as ammonia, increase in the body. The quantities of other substances, such as neurotransmitters, which are related to brain function, go

unchecked; therefore, many patients with cirrhosis develop prolonged confusion.

Esophageal Varices

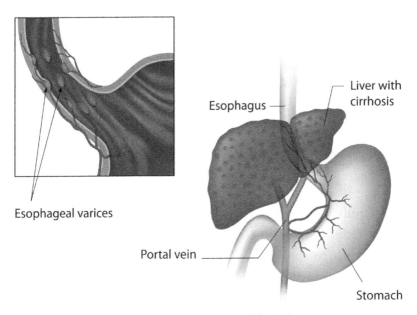

Esophagus

Liver with
cirrhosis

Esophageal varices

Portal vein

Stomach

Figure 12: Effect of "back pressure" of blood due to scarring
of the liver. (permission from fotosearch.com)

Helen was in the intensive care unit for the next few days. In
all, she needed five units of blood. Additionally, she was given
clotting factors, as well as platelets. She started to feel better over
next few days and began to eat a little. The doctors were still
monitoring Helen's blood count as she was transferred to the
step-down unit. Her abdomen had swollen up with fluid, and
she was complaining of belly distention and pain.

The liver produces albumin, a protein essential for circulation. The lack of albumin results in swelling of the body, and particularly in fluid collecting in the abdomen, which needs to be drained periodically. Patients complain of increasing weakness and a host of other problems. For many patients with alcoholism, infections with hepatitis B and hepatitis C viruses are an additional challenge. Patients with liver disease are deficient in vitamins, iron, electrolytes, and glucose stored in the body.

Four liters of fluid were drained from Helen's abdomen with a catheter through a needle. Even then, she was complaining of belly pain and asking for pain medications. She refused therapies, remained fairly weak, and was in no shape to go back home. The hospital made arrangements for Helen to go to a nursing home. At this time, the doctors talked to the patient and family about considerations for long-term care as well as resuscitation.

The daughters wanted to know, "What were Helen's chances?" As mentioned, advanced cirrhosis is mostly irreversible scarring of the liver. Patients who have mild cirrhosis may do well after quitting alcohol. Many such patients can experience reasonable long-term function.

Health-care teams use the model for end-stage liver disease (MELD) to assess the severity of cirrhosis and predict patient survival. The MELD score takes into account liver and kidney function. Helen's score was calculated at twenty-four. With such a score, Helen's chance of dying within three-months would be around 20 percent. Among patients who die, the cause is often infections of the fluid in the abdomen or somewhere else. Massive bleeding or prolonged confusion can also lead to demise. Multiorgan failure, including kidney failure, can add to the causes of death. Death can happen rather rapidly and sometimes out of the blue. Therefore, Helen had a one-in-five chance of having something happen to her and of dying within three months.

So then, is Helen's condition terminal? Gastroenterologists would be reluctant to call this patient terminal. They would continue to hope that the patient's condition could be optimized. They would like to see Helen refrain from alcohol and take prescribed medications. Then, once in stable condition, they would check the MELD score again to get a baseline. Doctors look at a biopsy, ultrasound or CT scan of the liver, and blood tests, as well as check the patient's medical history to determine the progression of the cirrhosis. Helen may have enough liver function to continue to survive with some limitations. Patients live with jaundice, recurring fluid accumulation in the abdomen, and bleeding that may require more banding. There is always some weakness and continued risk of periodic confusion. Many face increased risk of liver cancer.

Stomach doctors sometimes offer stent placement in the liver to reduce the pressures on the veins and reduce frequent bleeding. Some patients meet the criteria for a liver transplant. A transplant is not a solution for everyone; it requires commitment. Candidates must give up alcohol and go through physical, as well as psychological, testing to confirm that they are good candidates for transplant. Other responsibilities that transplant patients have to meet include monitoring, follow-up, and immune-suppression medications. A good support system helps. Patients with high MELD scores may be ranked higher on the transplant list. Many patients may die while waiting for a transplant, as only half of the patients in need receive one.

What if Helen's MELD score were forty? That would give her a three-month mortality rate of 71 percent. Would she be called terminal then? Should she choose comfort care at that stage? In this case, comfort care might mean not choosing aggressive modes such as transfusion and life support. It is a personal decision. The patient should consider the quality and enjoyment of his or her life, given the set of illnesses, before deciding on comfort care.

The CDC provide the Health-related Quality of Life Measure (HRQOL). Paraphrasing this five-component questionnaire, HRQOL includes the following:

1) How do you perceive your health: good or bad?
2) How has your physical health been over last thirty days?
3) How has your mental health been over last thirty days?
4) To what degree is your activity been limited by physical and mental health issues?
5) What is the number of days over the last thirty days that you have experienced pain performing usual activities, felt sad, felt depressed, felt worried or anxious, or didn't get enough rest or sleep?

The point is this: in any advanced irreversible illness with no scope for improvement, scoring low on the HRQOL may suggest the consideration of comfort care. Patients with advanced liver disease score poorly on HRQOL questions and report reduced quality of life.

Helen was so weak that she could not get out of bed without help. She would need to enter a nursing home, and the family wondered if she would ever reach her previous functioning level. She did not eat well enough to replenish her proteins, and it was clear to the doctors that recovery to stable cirrhosis was going to be a long and slow process. Helen said that she had been doing okay before all these events. Right now, she felt upset about everything and wanted to be left alone. She was focused on pain medications and did not want therapies or mobilization out of bed. Before coming into the hospital, Helen was helped by her friend, who cooked for her. She barely fed and bathed herself. The key to recovery is a strong desire to get better and effort in that direction, so Helen had a tough task ahead of her.

Even for patients who have relatively stable cirrhosis, life expectancy may be limited to nine to ten years. These patients do not qualify as terminal but rather as "limited-life-expectancy patients." Palliative care consultation is very appropriate for patients in Helen's condition.

Helen decided to remain on full support. She preferred to have CPR, blood transfusions, and dialysis if the doctors felt that they would help. She was later discharged to a nursing home.

Eighteen

What is the expectation from aggressive care?

Pauline was forty when her husband left her. This was particularly hard for her because she had never worked before. Her son seemed to have some mental challenges, and Pauline worried about him. With her husband gone, it was tough putting enough food on the table. Transport to and from work was also a problem. Pauline managed somehow with government help. Her sister was her only real support.

When Pauline was forty-five, she started to notice increased swelling in her face and legs. Thus, began her extended encounters with the medical system. Upon investigation, it was discovered that Pauline had weakened kidneys. Additionally, it turned out that she had diabetes and high blood pressure, likely the cause of her kidney problems. She was not surprised; her mother had those problems, too. The hospital's diabetes educator explained many things to her. Pauline had been having symptoms of diabetes for some time. Feeling thirsty all the time was one of them, although she was drinking soda pop when she shouldn't have. The diabetes educator gave Pauline multiple pamphlets and a sugar-checking machine, and showed Pauline how to prick herself and check her sugar level, but it was all too much. Just like that, unexpected, she was to manage a special diet and take pills. Would she afford it?

Kidneys remove excess water and waste from the body. One healthy kidney will do the job. Without kidneys, survival becomes impossible. Kidney failure can set in quickly in very ill patients due to poor circulation or toxins.

Kidney failure will occur with reduction of blood supply to the filtering complexes, the glomeruli. Diabetes, high cholesterol, and high blood pressure will make the supplying vessels thick, hard, and choked with plaques. A multitude of diseases, infections, immune problems (like lupus), and toxins can damage the glomeruli directly. Lastly, there can be many diseases affecting the collecting system of the urine, such as stones or cancers, which can block the kidneys and cause gradual or sudden loss of kidney function.

Advanced-stage kidney disease may not be manageable by medication and diet alone. Dialysis (mechanical filtering) of fluid and electrolytes may be required. Hemodialysis is a process of taking blood through a catheter placed in a vein into a dialysis machine. Usually, attachment to the machine is required three times a week for three hours each time. Often, a fistula, which is an artery-vein connection graft that allows for a large volume of blood flow as required for dialysis, is created surgically.

Pauline's challenges were many. She never had the financial or emotional capacity to manage her problems. She rarely controlled her sugar levels, and her blood pressure stayed consistently high. Her kidney function slowly declined over time, and by age 52, she required dialysis. A dialysis catheter was tunneled under her skin on her right chest. A catheter needs to be kept clean. Otherwise, it is frequently a source of infection.

Pauline hated dialysis but had no choice. Sometimes, though, there was no one to take her to the dialysis center, and she had to skip. Dialysis goes very well for patients who take due care, and they can have a relatively good quality of life. They may also be candidates for a kidney transplant. A transplant gives better longevity and function. Without a transplant, life expectancy is limited. In a fifty-year-old person, life expectancy may be eight to ten years. This number is an average; several governmental agencies put forth these numbers. Individuals in a difficult situation often don't manage well and end up in the hospital with a need for urgent dialysis because of fluid or toxin buildup.

Over the next few years, Pauline exhibited all the problems of poor dialysis. Fluid buildup in her body and lungs caused shortness of breath. Coronary artery disease, heart failure, and poor blood circulation to the legs bothered her. Abnormal deposits of calcium in her blood vessels had made her circulation even worse. Deposits of calcium in her skin were particularly painful to her. She had developed ulcers on her right toes that did not heal, ultimately requiring surgical removal of the toes. The itching of her skin was very bothersome, and nausea was common. Pauline was hopeful that the doctors would just give her pain medications. She was in bed often and on the couch much of the time. Pauline and her son had moved in with her sister.

One winter, at the age of sixty-two, Pauline was admitted to the hospital. Her blood pressure was very low, and she seemed slightly confused. She had missed her last several dialysis treatments since there was no one to take her. Her sister had been hospitalized and had been sick herself. Two months prior, Pauline had started to develop an ulcer on her left leg. After several appointments with the foot doctor, who had cleaned her wounds and arranged for dressing changes, the wound still appeared infected. Unfortunately, Pauline could not follow up with the foot doctor and had to call paramedics to bring her to the hospital because she was feeling sick.

The left leg now looked swollen, and foul-smelling pus was present in the wound. The skin was red and crackly all the way up to the middle of the leg. There was a concern for gas gangrene, an aggressive bacterial infection that requires emergency surgery. Surgeons said she might lose part of her leg. Pauline was overwhelmed. As it was, the removal of her right toes had made her life difficult. Losing her left leg would be devastating. But, the doctors were pushing her. Time for a decision was short and the surgery emergent. Doctors had placed an IV catheter—a "central line"—in Pauline's groin. Her blood pressure was low enough to require vasopressors.

Pauline's nephrologist whom she had known for many years and trusted, recommended she undergo surgery. As expected, she lost the left leg below the knee. The wound healing had been a problem because the skin was affected by calcium deposits known as *calciphylaxis*. The pain had become dominant. Pauline was not quite sure if she wanted to go on like this and wondered if she wanted any more dialysis. She would rather just have pain medications and comfort.

Pauline's albumin protein was low. The doctors did not think she would carry on like this for very long. Her mental clarity and ability to take care of herself were gone, and it meant she would have to move to a nursing home. Pauline was open to discussions with the palliative care team and indicated that she would talk to the team, but she could not make up her mind about whether she wanted to give up dialysis.

So, what causes death in patients with kidney failure? It is the usual suspects: heart disease, infection, stroke, multiorgan failure, and electrolyte imbalance. Long-term dialysis catheters are susceptible to infections. With coronary narrowing and peripheral vascular disease, organs fail easily. Patients who are malnourished and have dementia do very poorly. With a population that is growing older, the decision to start dialysis should be undertaken very carefully. Many calculators are available online, such as the one by QxMD, that predict the survival probability of a dialysis patients at six months. For Pauline, who was sixty-two, with low albumin and in poor condition, the chance that she would make it to six months was 50 percent. However, if she were having additional problems with her heart or developing multiorgan failure, she would die much sooner. It should be noted that all such calculators have significant limitations of accuracy for an individual prediction, though they are more accurate for a group.

Pauline's blood pressure stayed low, and she ended up at a long-term hospital instead of a nursing home. There, she could not get effective dialysis due to low blood pressure, even with supporting medications. Ultimately, due to significant lethargy and after family discussions, Pauline was transferred to hospice care.

Pauline's questions and fears at the end of life were understandable: I am being offered the dialysis to carry on. I do not know if the therapy is improving or changing my lifestyle.

———

Ron was diagnosed with what used to be called Wegener's granulomatosis, an autoimmune reaction against the cells of the small blood vessels resulting in vessel inflammation (vasculitis). The organs most commonly affected include the lungs and the kidneys. Ron had been coughing up blood one summer and then went into kidney failure at the age of sixty-nine. This illness resulted in prolonged hospitalization. Ron ended up on a breathing machine and then with a tracheostomy. He also needed long-term dialysis. Ultimately, Ron was placed on immune-suppression medications, liberated from the ventilator, and finally the tracheostomy tube was removed. The site healed, leaving a small scar.

Having a good access point for dialysis was a problem. Ron initially had a dialysis catheter placed in his neck veins, but had multiple problems with clotting and infection. A fistula for dialysis failed. Ultimately, he was left on peritoneal dialysis with an abdominal dialysis catheter.

The internal lining of the abdomen, called the *peritoneum*, can provide dialysis. It is called *peritoneal dialysis*. The process involves placement of a dialysis catheter into the abdomen. It is a slower and less efficient, but effective and a cheaper process. It affects the lifestyle of a patient differently, as it requires multiple exchanges of fluid in and out of the abdomen (Figure 13).

For a few years, Ron did better. He had difficulty with breathing and activity, but got around at home. His wife and daughter encouraged him and helped him with his twice-daily peritoneal dialysis exchanges. Ron's nephrologist followed him closely and saw him through multiple catheters, adjusted his immune medications, and performed innumerable tests.

Continuous ambulatory peritoneal dialysis

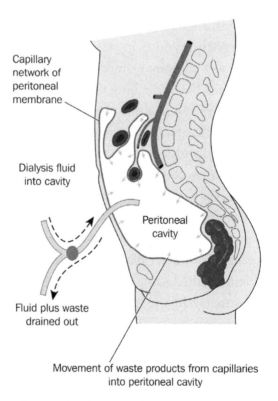

Figure 13: Peritoneal dialysis uses the abdominal cavity for electrolyte exchange. The process is slower and less effective than hemodialysis, but simpler and cheaper. (permission from fotosearch.com)

One day, after going through a bout of bronchitis, Ron presented to the hospital with breathing difficulty. He was now seventy-four years old and had been coughing constantly. His lungs sounded "full" as he periodically coughed up blood-tinged secretions. In his kidney tests, the levels of creatinine, potassium, and phosphorous were awry. Ron was retaining a lot more fluid compared with previous levels, mostly in the legs and lungs, so he was placed on high-flow oxygen and then ultimately on a BiPAP device to support his breathing. Ron was confused, occasionally agitated, and not taking in any food. The nurses placed a feeding tube down his nose. Peritoneal dialysis did not appear very affective, but the kidney physicians adjusted the dialysis fluid. Over the years Ron had become malnourished and debilitated with the vasculitis, immunosuppressive medications, and dialysis. Ron's progress in the hospital was minimal. There was no hope for Ron to go home. The only appropriate place for him was to a long-term hospital.

Ron was in the hospital for two weeks and then transferred to a long-term hospital, where he was in their intensive care unit setting. The vasculitis had left him with scarred and swollen lungs. His ability to bring up secretions was limited, requiring suctioning through a catheter down his nose. Unfortunately for Ron, he had a feeding tube going down the other nostril. The respiratory therapist additionally used a suction device to get rid of lingering phlegm in the back of the throat. For days, Ron had been on the BiPAP machine constantly. It became evident that he would need the breathing machine. The patient himself was not coherent. Much of the time, he was agitated and pulled at his restraints. Staff had given him pain and anxiety medications frequently, which didn't help the cycle of confusion.

Ron had now been in bed for three weeks, and he had a new skin breakdown. His wife and daughter, who were always at his bedside, saw the decline and wanted him on the ventilator. The doctors had a family meeting with all the children and wanted to know the goal of overall care, what the family expected out of the life support, and what they thought would happen over time. Ron's previous hospitalization many years before was etched in the memory of many family members. They thought he would fight his way back again. They wanted everything possible to be done. So, a breathing tube and then a tracheostomy tube were placed, and Ron was left on the ventilator.

The peritoneal dialysis was not very effective, and Ron was switched to regular hemodialysis through a temporary vein catheter. With aggressive hemodialysis, his fluid and electrolytes were better controlled, but the doctors at the long-term hospital could not liberate him from the breathing machine. At most, Ron would get off the breathing machine for a few hours; he then appeared fatigued, so was placed back on the ventilator. Ron occasionally recognized family, but much of the time he was restless. Over a period of six weeks, he had several courses of antibiotics and had suffered diarrhea.

Nutrition was still being supplied via the feeding tube through Ron's nose. Unfortunately, his nose was sore and bled multiple times. The doctors had not wanted to place a PEG-type surgical feeding tube without removing the abdominal peritoneal dialysis catheter. After much discussion among family and doctors, the peritoneal catheter was removed and a PEG was placed right into the stomach through the belly wall. Two days after starting tube feeding, Ron had a severe bout of infection, thought to be in the space around the stomach—*peritonitis*. He died two days later.

Ron's case exemplifies how we as a nation spend hundreds of thousands of dollars at the end of life. When providing aggressive care, the caregivers and patient/family must balance the risks and benefits of intervention and the possibility of survival against a level of enjoyment of life. Ron did not have any say in the situation. Many in the family would say they themselves would not want to go through this, but Ron was a fighter. They had seen him pull through before. Doctors did not want to place Ron on the ventilator, place another tracheostomy, perform hemodialysis, or place a feeding tube. They knew he was not going to do well. They could tell because of many things: mortality associated with vasculitis and kidney failure, the patient's age, malnutrition, delirium, and multiorgan failure at the time of discharge from the hospital to the long-term hospital. Mortality in such a case is extremely high. Would Ron have wanted this? He did not say it before his illness and could not say it during his illness.

Conclusion

Balancing Expectations

Balancing patient expectations is an important reason to record such stories. Patients and their families frequently go into an intensive care unit "blind." The subsequent decision process is confusing. The patients, and often the physicians, do not know the implications of prescribed therapies.

The majority of intensive care unit patients get better and move out of the ICU. The patients with long-term illnesses require readmission. Reduced functional capacity prior to hospital admission does not bode well for real long-term recovery. A big stroke, as in Florence's case, turns into a terminal event because of severe underlying COPD. Patients with a long-term illness are encouraged to understand their disease and to do their best to stay well. They are asked to think about the quality of life they enjoy. Whatever the decision for choosing or not choosing aggressive care, this book will hopefully help.

Medically speaking, there are different ways to quantify health and well-being. Many are discussed in this book. Factors, right or wrong, that affect patients and families in the choice of aggressive care are listed. Everyone should talk to the family about their desire for aggressive health care. Where do they draw the line? At which point in the spectrum of quality of life will they ask for palliation? A living will and DNR should be utilized much more frequently by patients in terminal condition. The truth is that they are doing themselves a favor, whatever they choose. The guidance to the family is invaluable.

Terminal and life-limiting conditions require patients to confront the possibility of death. Patients should undergo appropriate therapies, embrace new chemotherapy protocols, and consider newer technologies while at the same time maintaining realistic expectations. Particularly in terminal stages, if the decision is full code, then the *expectation of life must be balanced against the reality of prolonging death*. Palliative care and hospice services are helpful in supporting patients with life-limiting illness, *often improving quality of life and sometimes prolonging life*. Hospice does not mean giving up; patients can still undergo therapies.

Concerns regarding limiting aggressive care are also noted throughout the book. The inability of a patient to know and react to the future and the inability of doctors or scales to predict outcomes very accurately are the main concerns. There is fear that a DNR patient will get inadequate care, as well as anxiety regarding DNR discussions when families don't believe or hear the doctors. Such concerns benefit from these stories. It is hard to believe something that one has never seen or experienced. Many issues are mitigated by selecting proper level of care in a proper facility.

Young doctors can benefit from such stories. Can doctors predict what will happen in a week, a month, or a year? What do doctors expect their treatment is going to achieve for the patient? If their patient is terminal, are they forthright with him or her? After all, such discussions require additional time and emotional investment. It is *easier to just promise to try the next fix*. Can doctors identify subgroups of patients who are destined for short recovery or for death and tailor the treatments accordingly? Most intensive care unit doctors provide "episodes" of care; they are encouraged to follow patients through the long-term acute care hospital and nursing homes to understand the full spectrum of their interventions.

Balancing the expectations of health delivery models also becomes evident in these stories. Medicare and long-term acute care hospitals have a responsibility to disseminate the data of health outcomes. Such information is hard to find. Tracheotomy and feeding tubes allow discharge to a long-term acute care hospital quickly. Long term acute care hospital care is great for some patients and problematic for others.

Health-care advertisers should be circumspect. Performing high-technology procedures may not be the answer for all patients. Hospitals, specialty clinics, and drug companies do patients a disservice by creating an impression that everything can be fixed by modern medicine.

Selecting the right patients for aggressive care is important for patient survival and community resources. The correct selection allows physicians to meet the expectations of recovery.

In conclusion, my hope is that this book serves its purpose of providing the "big picture" on the recovery of the very sick, allowing pertinent discussions on the goals of care. The book should induce one to create advanced directives. Perhaps the most important component to these discussions is the attitude towards death. The secret may be "being ready." I did not dwell on this much but mention in Naru's as well as in Florence's stories. They both said they had enjoyed their lives and were left with no further wishes. I will mention the words of our vivacious, intelligent, and beautiful nurse practitioner, whom we lost to cancer. A few days before she passed away in hospice, she talked about confronting death. With tears in her bright eyes and a smile on her face she said, "Dr. Thakore, I am at peace."

Further Reading

In this age of *Wikipedia*, information of all kinds is at our fingertips—literally. And while *Wikipedia* can be a useful resource, it is far from being the only one. Below you will find a list of suggested websites selected for their accessible information that expands on and enhances the issues and topics addressed in this book.

I have *no* affiliation or association with any of the organizations or businesses cited. The sole purpose of suggesting these pages is their relevance and usefulness to readers of this book. The links have been grouped by chapter heading. Please use your own judgment when visiting these sites.

All the sites can be accessed through a single page with all these links. Once you are on that page, you can get to all the further reading sites with a single click: http://www.pulm-care.com/thakore.html.

Introduction
Life expectancy and leading causes of death:
Joaquin Vu et al. *National Vital Statistics Report* 64, no. 2 (2016).
http://www.cdc.gov/nchs/data/nvsr/nvsr64/nvsr64_02.pdf

End of life information:
US Department of Health and Human Services, National Institute of Aging, "End of Life: Helping with Comfort and Care."
https://www.nia.nih.gov/health/publication/end-life-helping-comfort-and-care/introduction

Chapter 1
Illinois advance directives:
Illinois Department of Public Health website. "Advance Directives."
http://www.dph.illinois.gov/topics-services/health care-regulation/nursing-homes/advance-directives

Illinois living will (document):
Illinois Department of Health website
http://www.dph.illinois.gov/sites/default/files/forms/living-will-040416.pdf

Ohio living will and health care power of attorney (documents):
Ohio Hospital Association
http://ohiohospitals.org/OHA/media/Images/Membership%20Services/Documents/advance-directives-2015-update-final5.pdf

Problems with the living will:
Angela Fagerlin and Carl E. Schneider. 2004. Enough: The Failure of the Living Will. *Hastings Center Report* 34, no. 2 (2004): 30–42. http://www.thehastingscenter.org/pdf/publications/hcr_mar_apr_2004_enough.pdf

Aging:
Mayo Clinic website, "Aging: What to expect" http://www.mayoclinic.org/healthy-lifestyle/healthy-aging/in-depth/aging/art-20046070

National Institutes of Health, National Library of Medicine website, "Aging changes in organs - tissue - cells" https://www.nlm.nih.gov/medlineplus/ency/article/004012.htm

Chapter 2
Cardiac arrest information for families:
Mayo Clinic website, "Sudden cardiac arrest" http://www.mayoclinic.org/diseases-conditions/sudden-cardiac-arrest/symptoms-causes/dxc-20164872

Cardio-pulmonary resuscitation (CPR)
American Heart Association website, "Cardiac Arrest vs Heart Attack" http://cpr.heart.org/AHAECC/CPRAndECC/AboutCPRFirstAid/CardiacArrestvsHeartAttack/UCM_473213_Cardiac-Arrest-vs-Heart-Attack.jsp

Sue Maynard Campbell, a champion for people with disabilities: Sian Vasey. Sue Maynard Campbell. *The Guardian.* June 2008. http://www.theguardian.com/society/2008/jun/16/disability

Chapter 3
Some facts on ALS:
ALS website
http://www.alsa.org/about-als/facts-you-should-know.html

Chapter 4
Older drivers:
Centers for Disease Control and Prevention (CDC) website. National Center for Injury Prevention and Control, Division of Unintentional Injury Prevention, "Older Adult Drivers"
http://www.cdc.gov/motorvehiclesafety/older_adult_drivers/

"Do not resuscitate" (DNR) order:
National Institutes of Health, National Library of Medicine, "Do-not-resuscitate order"
Updated by Laura J. Martin, MD, February 6, 2016.
https://www.nlm.nih.gov/medlineplus/ency/patientinstructions/000473.htm

Information and statistics on disability
Centers for Disease Control and Prevention (CDC) website
http://www.cdc.gov/ncbddd/disabilityandhealth/

Function evaluation
Mahoney, F. I., and D. Barthel. Functional evaluation: the
Barthel Index. *Maryland State Med Journal* 14 (1965):56–61.
Used with permission.
http://www.strokecenter.org/wp-content/uploads/2011/08/
barthel.pdf

Chapter 5
Useful information on coma scales:
Brainline.org website, "What is the Glasgow Coma Scale?"
http://www.brainline.org/content/2010/10/what-is-the-glasgow-
coma-scale.html

Traumatic brain injury (TBI):
Nucleus Medical Media, "Concussion/Traumatic Brain Injury
(TBI)"
Published by Nucleushealth.com (2012)
https://www.youtube.com/watch?v=55u5Ivx31og

IMPACT.org, International Mission for Prognosis and Analysis
of Clinical Trials in TBI
http://www.tbi-impact.org/

Deep venous thrombosis:
Mayo Clinic website, "Deep vein thrombosis (DVT)"
http://www.mayoclinic.org/diseases-conditions/deep-vein-
thrombosis/basics/treatment/con-20031922

Chapter 6

The problem of delirium in intensive care unit patients: intensive care unit Delirium and Cognitive Impairment Study Group website
http://www.icudelirium.org/patients.html

Description of the brain injury known as a subdural hematoma: Harvard Medical School, Patient Education Center, "Subdural Hematoma"
http://www.patienteducationcenter.org/articles/subdural-hematoma/

Chapter 7

Multiorgan failure:
Posted by ABD broadcast, Australia. "Multiple Organ Failure." August 7, 2014.
http://www.aABD.net.au/catalyst/stories/4060404.htm

Mortality scoring:
Breslow, M. J., and O. Badawi. Severity Scoring in the Critically Ill: Part 1—Interpretation and Accuracy of Outcome Prediction Scoring Systems. *Chest* 141, no. 1 (2012): 245-252, doi: 10.1378/chest.11-0330.
http://journal.publications.chestnet.org/article.aspx?articleid=1149018

SOFA calculator:
QxMD website, Sequential Organ Failure Assessment (SOFA)

https://qxmd.com/calculate/calculator_268/sequential-organ-failure-assessment-sofa

Chapter 8
Stroke information:
National Stroke Association website
http://www.stroke.org/

Stroke, severity, and outcome:
Ellis, Mary Ellen, and Erica Cirino. "Massive Stroke: Symptoms, Treatments, and Outlook." 2016. Medically reviewed by Graham Rogers, MD, Healthline.
http://www.healthline.com/health/stroke/massive-stroke#Overview1

Chapter 9
Opioid abuse:
Volkow, Nora D. "America's Addiction to Opioids: Heroin and Prescription Drug Abuse." National Institute on Drug Abuse. NIH. 2014.
https://www.drugabuse.gov/about-nida/legislative-activities/testimony-to-congress/2016/americas-addiction-to-opioids-heroin-prescription-drug-abuse

Legal thinking and the history of withdrawal of care:
Luce, John, and Ann Alpers. Legal Aspects of Withholding and Withdrawing Life Support from Critically Ill Patients in the

United States and Providing Palliative Care to Them. *American Journal of Respiratory and Critical Care Medicine* 162, no. 6(2000):2029–2032, doi: 10.1164/ajrccm.162.6.1-00
http://www.atsjournals.org/doi/full/10.1164/ajrccm.162.6.1-00#.V0w9WNLmpYc

Withdrawal of ventilator, information for families:
American Association of Critical Care Nurses website, "Ventilator Withdrawal Guidelines."
http://www.aacn.org/WD/Palliative/Docs/mgh8.pdf

Chapter 10
Cancer:
American Cancer Society website
http://www.cancer.org/

Early palliative care in advanced cancers improves quality of life and extends life:
Howie, Lynn, and Jeffrey Peppercorn. Early palliative care in cancer treatment: rationale, evidence and clinical implications. *Therapeutic Advances in Medical Oncology* 5, no. 6 (2013): 318–323, doi: 10.1177/1758834013500375
http://www.ncbi.nlm.nih.gov/pmc/articles/PMC3799294/

End of life issues:
Howard LeWine, MD, Chief Medical Editor. "As cancer death approaches, palliative care may improve quality of life." Internet Publishing, Harvard Health Publications. Posted July 11, 2012.

http://www.health.harvard.edu/blog/as-cancer-death-approaches-palliative-care-may-improve-quality-of-life-201207115017

Chapter 11

Autoimmune disease:
Julie Roddick. "Autoimmune Disease." Medically reviewed by Steven Kim, MD, Healthline. July 22, 2015.
http://www.healthline.com/health/autoimmune-disorders#Overview1

Pulmonary hypertension:
Cleveland Clinic website, "What is pulmonary hypertension?" http://my.clevelandclinic.org/health/diseases_conditions/hic_pulmonary_hypertension_causes_symptoms_diagnosis_treatment

End of life issues:
PBS. Frontline. "Facing Death" PBS.org. November 2010.
http://www.pbs.org/wgbh/pages/frontline/facing-death/

Chapter 12

Pulmonary fibrosis:
National Institutes of Health, Health Topics, "Living with Idiopathic Pulmonary Fibrosis."
http://www.nhlbi.nih.gov/health/health-topics/topics/ipf/livingwith

Stephanie Pierce. "The Outlook for Idiopathic Pulmonary Fibrosis: Prognosis and Life Expectancy." Medically reviewed by George Krucik, MD, MBA. August 28, 2015
http://www.healthline.com/health/idiopathic-pulmonary-fibro-sis/outlook-for-ipf-prognosis-life-expectancy#1

Chapter 13
There are many reliable sites for information on coma and veg-etative state; check Brainline.org.

Ariel Sharon biography:
Biography.com Editors. "Ariel Sharon Biography." The Biography.com website. A&E Television Networks. August 24, 2016.
http://www.biography.com/people/ariel-sharon-9480655#early-life

Chapter 14
Chronic obstructive pulmonary disease (COPD):
COPD Foundation website
http://www.copdfoundation.org/

Late-stage COPD care:
Weiss, Barry D. Hospice Eligibility for Patients with COPD. *Elder Care.* 2010. (Updated May 2015.)
https://nursingandhealth.asu.edu/sites/default/files/hospice-care-for-copd.pdf

Foley catheter and infections: frequently asked questions:
CDC.gov, "FAQs about 'Catheter-Associated Urinary Tract Infection'"
http://www.cdc.gov/hai/pdfs/uti/CA-UTI_tagged-BW.pdf

Chapter 15
Robin Williams:
Smith, Nigel M. Robin Williams' widow: "It was not depression" that killed him. *The Guardian.* November 2015.
https://www.theguardian.com/film/2015/nov/03/robin-williams-disintegrating-before-suicide-widow-says

Alzheimer's disease:
Alzheimer's Association website
http://www.alz.org/

Chapter 16
Heart failure:
Ashley, E. A., and J. Niebauer. Cardiology Explained. London: Remedica. 2004. Chapter 7, "Heart Failure."
http://www.ncbi.nlm.nih.gov/books/NBK2218/

Classification of heart failure:
American Heart Association website, "Classes of Heart Failure."
http://www.heart.org/HEARTORG/Conditions/HeartFailure/AboutHeartFailure/Classes-of-Heart-Failure_UCM_306328_Article.jsp#.V05CP9Lmpjo

Heart failure and palliative care:
Adler, Eric D., Judith Z. Goldfinger, Jill Kalman, Michelle E. Park, and Diane E. Meier. Palliative Care in the Treatment of Advanced Heart Failure. *Circulation* 120, no. 25 (2009):2597–2606.
http://dx.doi.org/10.1161/CIRCULATIONAHA.109.869123
http://circ.ahajournals.org/content/120/25/2597.full
(Important article: Palliative care is not hospice. Palliative care prolongs life and improves symptoms)

Chapter 17
Cirrhosis:
Jeffrey A Gunter, MD. "Cirrhosis Overview." Reviewed 1/4/2016.
emedicinehealth.com
http://www.emedicinehealth.com/cirrhosis/article_em.htm#cirrhosis_overview

MELD calculator:
MDcalc.com. MELD Score (Model for End-Stage Liver Disease) (12 and older)
http://www.mdcalc.com/meld-score-model-for-end-stage-liver-disease-12-and-older/

Transition of care for patients with end-stage liver disease:
Cox-North, Paula, et al. The Transition to End-of-Life Care in End-Stage Liver Disease. *Journal of Hospice & Palliative Nursing* 15, no. 4(2013):209–215, doi: 10.1097/NJH.0b013e318289f4b0.
http://journals.lww.com/jhpn/Pages/articleviewer.aspx?year=2013&issue=06000&article=00005&type=Fulltext

Chapter 18

Kidney facts, prevention, and other information:
National Kidney Foundation website
https://www.kidney.org/prevention

Mortality in renal failure calculator:
Qxmd.com. Estimated six-month mortality on dialysis (calculator).
https://www.qxmd.com/calculate/calculator_135/6-month-mortality-on-hd

Conclusion:

Balancing expectations:
Benson, W. F., and N. Aldrich. Advance Care Planning: Ensuring Your Wishes Are Known and Honored If You Are Unable to Speak for Yourself. Critical Issue Brief. Centers for Disease Control and Prevention. 2012. www.cdc.gov/aging.
http://www.cdc.gov/aging/pdf/advanced-care-planning-critical-issue-brief.pdf

About the Author

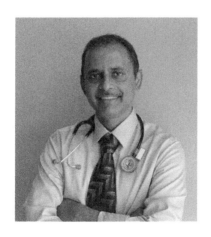

G nan Thakore, MD, has been working in intensive care for twenty-five years. He currently serves as the director of the ICU at Miami Valley Hospital in Dayton, Ohio. Thakore studied at Brown University and now passes his knowledge on to the next generation as an associate clinical professor of medicine at the Boonshoft School of Medicine at Wright State University in Dayton. He is married and has two grown children.